As One Lives, So One Dies

Werner Gross

As One Lives, So One Dies

On the Life and Death of Great Psychotherapists

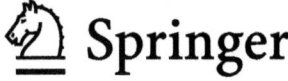

Werner Gross
Psychologische Praxis
Gelnhausen, Hessen, Germany

ISBN 978-3-662-70060-0   ISBN 978-3-662-70061-7   (eBook)
https://doi.org/10.1007/978-3-662-70061-7

Translation from the German language edition: "Wie man lebt, so stirbt man" by Werner Gross, © Der/die Herausgeber bzw. der/die Autor(en), exklusiv lizenziert an Springer-Verlag GmbH, DE, ein Teil von Springer Nature 2021. Published by Springer Berlin Heidelberg. All Rights Reserved.

This book is a translation of the original German edition "Wie man lebt, so stirbt man" by Werner Gross, published by Springer-Verlag GmbH, DE in 2021. The translation was done with the help of an artificial intelligence machine translation tool. A subsequent human revision was done primarily in terms of content, so that the book will read stylistically differently from a conventional translation. Springer Nature works continuously to further the development of tools for the production of books and on the related technologies to support the authors.

© The Editor(s) (if applicable) and The Author(s), under exclusive license to Springer-Verlag GmbH, DE, part of Springer Nature 2024

This work is subject to copyright. All rights are solely and exclusively licensed by the Publisher, whether the whole or part of the material is concerned, specifically the rights of translation, reprinting, reuse of illustrations, recitation, broadcasting, reproduction on microfilms or in any other physical way, and transmission or information storage and retrieval, electronic adaptation, computer software, or by similar or dissimilar methodology now known or hereafter developed.
The use of general descriptive names, registered names, trademarks, service marks, etc. in this publication does not imply, even in the absence of a specific statement, that such names are exempt from the relevant protective laws and regulations and therefore free for general use.
The publisher, the authors and the editors are safe to assume that the advice and information in this book are believed to be true and accurate at the date of publication. Neither the publisher nor the authors or the editors give a warranty, expressed or implied, with respect to the material contained herein or for any errors or omissions that may have been made. The publisher remains neutral with regard to jurisdictional claims in published maps and institutional affiliations.

Illustration: (c) rolffimages/stock.adobe.com

This Springer imprint is published by the registered company Springer-Verlag GmbH, DE, part of Springer Nature.
The registered company address is: Heidelberger Platz 3, 14197 Berlin, Germany

If disposing of this product, please recycle the paper.

Preface: Prologue

The living close the eyes of the dead. The dead open the eyes of the living. (Slavic Proverb)

"Practice dying," Plato is said to have stated on his deathbed when a friend asked him to summarize his life's work in one sentence.

Until the present day, philosophers have dealt with death and dying in their works. Some even believe that philosophizing means nothing more than learning to die. Despite the countless scientific findings—death remains a mystery and a taboo. We will all not escape it and will experience it at some point. And whether scientific "head knowledge" helps and provides security for the preparation for these last conscious moments is at least questionable. A religious cynic once said: "Keep bread away from mice—and scientists from the soul."

But no matter how many medical insights we gather about our last seconds or minutes, no matter how many "near-death experiences" we document, research, read and discuss—the uncertainty will probably remain in the future. Some may have stood on the threshold and looked into the dark abyss (or into the dazzling light). They may have also jumped or fallen—but no one who was truly dead has returned. We know at best the first stages of dying—not death.

However, many people do not want to accept this. Especially when they fall into emotional crises or emotional turbulence, there is an (apparent) inherent tendency in humans to want to psychologically explain and understand this mystery. Because dealing with death and dying is part of the canon of great philosophical fundamental questions:

- Who am I?
- Where do I come from?
- Where am I going?
- How will I die?
- What is the purpose of my life?
- What am I supposed to do here? What is my task?
- What do I want to do with my life?
- What is important to me in life?

These are rather **philosophical** (or religious) questions. The **psychology** rather asks:

Why, how, and through what have I become the way I am? What of it can be changed? Am I truly "the architect of my own fortune" or just the executor of the genes inherent in me—or of the fate assigned to me? And with what must I (like it or not) live?

After all, this involves questions of personality structure (formerly called character), satisfaction, and happiness:

Have I just grown old or have I understood something? Have I just cunningly made my way through life? Or have I also become a bit wise in life? Do you have to understand life—or is it enough to find your way in it?

Above all, psychotherapy as a medical treatment often expands on these questions. After all, many psychotherapy patients ask themselves: Why have I become mentally or physically ill? Am I responsible for what I have done with my life so far (according to the motto: "it's my own fault")? Or am I simply a victim of genetic, familial, or societal circumstances? Which crises have I not adequately coped with? Or have I simply strayed too far from my predetermined path and ended up in a dead end in the thicket of unpredictable life with its confusions and complications, from which I can no longer find my way out without the help of psychotherapy (or off-the-shelf meaning systems, such as those offered by religions)?

Essentially, these questions have to do with the fact that we as humans are highly malleable by what happens to us over the course of our lives—unfortunately, also deformable.

Unlike other living beings on this planet, we humans are ultimately "physiological preterm births", who are thrown into this world much more unfinished and vulnerable. A dog, a cat, a horse naturally also need the protection, care, and food of their parents and their environment after birth—but they are able to move away from their parents and explore the world shortly after birth.

We humans are much more unfinished and dependent on a benevolent direct environment—namely: mother, father, family. We need a "social womb" that protects us and shapes us, molds us and allows us to mature. This environment can be positive by promoting the abilities inherent in us and helping to develop them, but we are also much more drastically **mis**shaped by upbringing and dramatic life events. And of course, this does not only apply to early childhood, but this fundamental vulnerability accompanies us throughout our lives—even if we do not like to acknowledge it.

How we deal with the challenges of life (learn), that determines our mental strength or weakness. (On the other hand, perhaps the development of our brain has exactly to do with this sensitivity and vulnerability, because our brain is a lifelong construction site that never gets finished—but that's a completely different topic …)

Because—the more severe the everyday downfalls, the injuries and deformations that life imposes and inflicts on us (or that we ourselves—e.g. through wrong decisions—produce), the closer we get to seeking support. In today's times, this is usually psychotherapy. What used to be priests, shamans, medicine men or gurus in other cultures, are (at least in our cultural circle) nowadays psychologists and psychotherapists. This relatively young profession is therefore attributed all sorts of—more or less magical—abilities by the general population. They are supposed to help us understand these everyday downfalls, process them, pull us out of this swamp of everyday life and get us fit again for the struggle of life—especially in these uncertain times after a pandemic.

In this context, there are a multitude of psychotherapeutic schools that have developed very different paths and strategies to help us understand who we are, how we got into this situation—and how we can get out again.

These psychotherapy schools usually trace back to a founding figure—sometimes even to several. However, psychologists and psychotherapists often know little about the lives of the founders of the psychotherapy schools, whose methods they work with. Many do not even know how these founders lived, what trials and tribulations they went through in their lives, what crises they experienced and how they overcame them. What lifestyle ultimately emerged from this—and what does this lifestyle have to do with the psychotherapy method and the theory they developed? Are there striking events and experiences—and do these find their reflection in the development of the psychotherapy method (e.g., Freud, his throat cancer, and the postulation of the "Destrudo", death drive, as a counterpoint to the life energy "Libido")? And finally, how did they die? Is there a connection between lifestyle, style of dying, and psychotherapy method?

For without a doubt, there are a number of psychotherapists, doctors, and psychologists who have left their distinctive mark on psychotherapy—this healing method that is still quite young compared to other medical faculties. In a very special way, these are of course the founders of psychotherapy schools: Sigmund Freud (psychoanalysis), Alfred Adler (individual psychology) or Carl Gustav Jung (analytical psychology). But also the thoughts of Jacob L. Moreno, the founder of psychodrama, Fritz Perls (Gestalt therapy), Wilhelm Reich (body psychotherapeutic methods), Karlfried Graf Dürckheim (initiatic therapy) and Nossrat Peseschkian (positive psychotherapy) still leave their traces in the psychotherapeutic and psychological cosmos today. As great as their ideas were—the great psychologists also died humanly in their time. After all: No one escapes life alive.

No question: There are lifestyles, that is, the individual way in which someone designs their life—more or less consciously. No one will doubt that this **lifestyle**—at least in part—can be influenced willingly. Certainly, this lifestyle is not consistently the same, it is related to a person's personality structure and can vary from life phase to life phase—also depending on what has happened to the individual person in life ("life events") and how they have learned to deal with it. However—the basic patterns often remain.

But is there also something like a **style of dying**, that is, the predetermined way in which someone dies? And: Can it be deliberately influenced or are we more or less at the mercy of this process? And is there a connection between lifestyle and style of dying? Does the lifestyle have an influence on how someone dies? Or is it the result of a certain lifestyle, for which one essentially gets the bill?

I have been dealing with these questions repeatedly since the mid-1980s. And it all started quite unspectacularly. I remember it very clearly, even though it's been quite a while: It was on an unusually hot Sunday for May. We were lying on a meadow near a small village in the Hessian Vogelsberg. The bees were buzzing, the butterflies were fluttering, the brook was babbling idyllically. It was almost windless, only a few cirrus clouds were quietly evaporating in the sky and the sun was burning. We had just had a small picnic, were relaxing, reading and dozing off, when my partner said: "You have a strangely irregular mole on your back. A doctor should take a look at it."

At first, I didn't think much of it, especially since my partner often reacted hypersensitively to all sorts of minor changes and tended to take minor ailments overly seriously.

But something inside me wouldn't let me rest. So, a few days later, I really went to my dermatologist. When he shook his head thoughtfully and said, "This really doesn't look good. We need to send this in," I was stunned. In that week, until the results of the examination came from the lab, my inner carousel started to spin. At night, I woke up drenched in sweat and startled from crazy dreams, with all sorts of absurd disease progressions, surgeries, and funerals.

Illness and death suddenly became something that was not only associated with other people—especially patients—but also with myself. My own somnambulistic certainty and the feeling of invulnerability were lost. Not only had the professional everyday life become leaden, but private life was also tough, laborious, and I constantly felt slightly dizzy. I had the feeling that a boomerang had hit me in the back of the head and I had a mild concussion. It was like a rendezvous with my fate.

During this time, I had already completed my training as a psychotherapist some years ago. And of course, illness, dying, and death had also been topics in my self-experience and self-analysis, but suddenly they took on a whole new intensity and seriousness. It was as if I had learned many theoretical concepts about swimming and had extensively practiced dry swimming—but suddenly, through this experience, I was pushed into the water and now had to see how I could get my head above the waterline again without losing sight of my goal and continue swimming swiftly.

I had just opened a small private practice in Frankfurt, but I was also still working as a journalist and publicist. And I was particularly interested in the topic of what the real differences are between the various schools of psychotherapy—not only in terms of the methods and techniques they use, but also the theoretical foundations on which they are based—so: philosophy, image of humanity, concept of illness, therapy goals, etc.

So I inevitably came to the people who founded the psychotherapy schools. What kind of people were they? How did they come to develop their method? What confusions and complications did they go through in their lives? How did they overcome these? What of this has found its reflection in the psychotherapy methods?

And I had a special connection to each of the individuals and their methods presented in this book.

Thus, as a psychologist and psychotherapist, I have dealt with the life and death of great psychotherapists, perhaps with the (more or less conscious) question: What can I learn from this for myself and my life, but also for my profession?

So, I have studied the life and death of Freud, Jung, Adler, and other psychotherapists, and where possible, conducted interviews—with the founders of psychotherapy schools (if they were still alive), with their children, and with close female and male students who have personally worked with them.

And that's where my second profession as a journalist and publicist came to my aid. During this time, I—in addition to publishing books—primarily worked for various public broadcasting stations (Hessischer Rundfunk, Südwestfunk, WDR, Deutsche Welle, Radio Bremen …) and mainly prepared and produced psychological topics for cultural and scientific programs. In this way, I was able to win over several editorial teams for the topic of death and dying of the great psychotherapists and thus also conduct interviews with:

- Karlfried Graf Dürckheim (initiatic therapy) in Todtmoos/Rütte.
- Alexandra and Kurt Adler (the two children of Alfred Adler), who practiced in New York.
- Marie Louise von Franz, a direct student of C. G. Jung, in Kuesnacht on Lake Zurich.
- Hamid Peseschkian, the son of Nossrat Peseschkian, who founded positive psychotherapy, was available for a conversation. (I myself had almost 10 years of contact with Nossrat Peseschkian, which ultimately persuaded me—after all my various trainings—to also complete the training as a positive psychotherapist, so that I have now become an international master trainer of positive psychotherapy.)
- In addition to my training in depth psychology and psychoanalysis, I am also a psychodramatist, and naturally, I wanted to get to know Jacob L. Moreno better. To do this, Gretel Leutz, a direct student of Jacob L. Moreno and head of the Moreno Institute Überlingen, was willing to be interviewed.
- And since I had a lot of Gestalt therapeutic self-therapy and self-experience behind me, I was naturally also interested in the life of Fritz Perls.
- In addition, I am also a body psychotherapist myself and Wilhelm Reich is considered the forefather of all depth psychologically based body psychotherapeutic methods. Therefore, it was clear that I would also engage with his life.

In the confrontation with the life stories and the method of various psychotherapists and the way they lived and died, the question always arose: What of this have I incorporated into my psychotherapeutic work—and what has remained distant to me? Which methods suit me—and which do not?

But there was something else: I wanted to find out if there is not only a connection between lifestyle and style of dying, but also whether the development of the psychotherapy method is somehow linked to it …

Thus, the aim of this book is to convey knowledge about the life and death of great psychotherapists—and what it has to do with the development of their psychotherapy method.

And is the implicit thesis correct that there is a connection between personal lifestyle, the style of dying, and the development of the respective psychotherapy method?

Quite apart from that, the general engagement with the topic of life, death, and dying is something that interests most of us—regardless of any psychotherapists—(or at least should interest us). There are one or two thoughts on these general questions in the respective transition chapters ("Interlude"). Even though we like to suppress it, the hidden question emerges: What will it be like for me? How will I probably die?

I enjoy reading what you think about it. Write to me: eMail: pfo-mail@t-online.de

Gelnhausen, in Autumn/Winter 2021   Werner Gross

Contents

1 Sigmund Freud (1856–1939): The Morphine-Dulled Pain of Dying   1
- 1.1 Childhood and Youth   3
- 1.2 Studies   4
- 1.3 Josef Breuer   4
- 1.4 Martha Bernays—Starting a Family   5
- 1.5 Cocaine   5
- 1.6 Charcot and Hypnosis   6
- 1.7 From Physiology to Psychology   6
- 1.8 Cathartic Method   7
- 1.9 Wilhelm Fließ   7
- 1.10 Free Association and Couch   7
- 1.11 Psychoanalysis   8
- 1.12 Sexuality   8
- 1.13 Self-analysis: Where Id was, Ego shall be   8
- 1.14 Psychoanalytic Movement   9
- 1.15 Marriage and Family   9
- 1.16 Physical Constitution and Diseases   9
- 1.17 Libido and Destrudo   10
- 1.18 The Destruction of the Life's Work   11
- 1.19 Exile in London   12
- 1.20 Euthanasia Morphine   12
- 1.21 Sapere aude   13

1.22	The Third Great Humiliation of Humanity	13
1.23	Conclusion	14
Further Reading		14

2 Interlude I: On Aging — 15
2.1	Wisdom in Old Age—Senility—Stubbornness in Old Age	16
2.2	Three Types of Age	17
2.3	Review	17
Further Reading		18

3 Alfred Adler (1870–1937): Sudden Death During a Walk — 19
3.1	Childhood and First Illnesses	21
3.2	Family Situation	22
3.3	School, Studies, and Start of Career	23
3.4	Starting a Family	23
3.5	Freud—Adler	24
3.6	Setting Variables	24
3.7	Separation	25
3.8	Individual Psychology	25
3.9	Compensation Ability	26
3.10	Unconscious Life Plan	27
3.11	Community Feeling and Life Goal	27
3.12	Activities	27
3.13	Educational Counseling Centers and Children's Clinics	28
3.14	Adler's Image of Humanity	28
3.15	Educational Ideas in "Red Vienna"	29
3.16	Publications and Lecture Tours	30
3.17	Relocation to the USA	30
3.18	Last Days	31
3.19	Cremation and Honorary Grave in Vienna	32
3.20	The Social Genius	32
3.21	Conclusion	32
Bibliography		33
Further Reading		33

4 Interlude II: On Dying — 35
4.1	Death as the Great Equalizer	36
4.2	A Fairy Tale	36
Further Reading		37

5	**Wilhelm Reich (1897–1957): Destruction of a Heretic**		39
	5.1	Emotional Illiterates	41
	5.2	"Emotional Plague"	41
	5.3	Inner World Pollution	42
	5.4	Libido Theory	42
	5.5	Childhood and Youth	43
	5.6	Psychoanalysis	44
	5.7	The Function of the Orgasm	45
	5.8	Psychoanalysis and Marxism	45
	5.9	Character Analysis	46
	5.10	Emigration	46
	5.11	Orgone I	47
	5.12	From Libido to Bioenergy	47
	5.13	Armorings	48
	5.14	Practice	48
	5.15	Physiology and Psychology	48
	5.16	Orgone Therapy	49
	5.17	Scandinavia—USA	50
	5.18	Savior	50
	5.19	Orgon II	50
	5.20	Einstein	51
	5.21	Charlatanism and Persecution	51
	5.22	Destruction of the Life's Work	52
	5.23	Prison and Death	52
	5.24	Conclusion	53
	Bibliography		53
6	**Interlude III: The Phases of Dying**		55
	6.1	Denial	56
	6.2	Anger	56
	6.3	Bargaining	56
	6.4	Depression	56
	6.5	Acceptance	57
	6.6	Individuality	57
	Further Reading		58
7	**Jacob Levy Moreno (1889–1974): "Playing God" or Directing Until the Last Scene**		59
	7.1	Birth—Truth(s) and Poetry	61
	7.2	Religious Influences	61
	7.3	Name Changes	61

7.4		Religious Maturity	62
7.5		Working with Marginalized Groups	62
7.6		Sociometry	62
7.7		Literary Avant-Garde	63
7.8		Impromptu Theater	63
7.9		Emigration to the USA	64
7.10		From Impromptu Play to Psychodrama	64
7.11		Taking Responsibility with the Action Method	65
7.12		Psychodrama: Approaches	65
7.13		Psychodrama: Procedure	66
7.14		Psychodrama: Roles	66
7.15		Psychodrama: Techniques	67
7.16		Psychodrama: Precursors	69
7.17		Stabilization	69
7.18		Publications	69
7.19		Beacon Hill Sanatorium and Moreno Institute	69
7.20		International Recognition	70
7.21		Women and Family	70
7.22		Daily Routine and Personality	71
7.23		The Wise Elder	72
7.24		Starvation?	73
7.25		Directing Until the Last Scene	75
7.26		Conclusion	77
		Further Reading	77
8	**Interlude IV: Types of Death and Styles of Dying**		**79**
	8.1	Definition and Transitions	80
	8.2	Natural and Unnatural Causes of Death	80
	8.3	Taboo Topic	81
	8.4	Classification and Philosophical Interpretation	81
		Further Reading	82
9	**Fritz Perls (1893–1970): "You Will Not Tell Me What to Do"**		**83**
	9.1	Education	84
	9.2	Exile	85
	9.3	Gestalt Therapy	85
	9.4	Human Potential Movement	86
	9.5	Image of Humanity	86
	9.6	Philosophy	87
	9.7	Publications and Esalen	87

9.8	Restlessness and Impatience	88
9.9	Gestalt Prayer	88
9.10	Awareness, Here and Now, and Growth	88
9.11	Freud and Perls	89
9.12	Gestalt Therapy and Gestalt Psychology: Foundations	89
9.13	Sources of Gestalt Therapy	90
9.14	Psychoanalysis	90
9.15	Gestalt Psychology	91
9.16	Behaviorism	91
9.17	Psychodrama	92
9.18	Zen Buddhism	92
9.19	Existentialism and Phenomenology	92
9.20	Wisdom of the Organism	93
9.21	Practice	94
9.22	Gestalt Kibbutz	95
9.23	Restlessness	95
9.24	Illness and Death	96
9.25	Dance of Death	96
9.26	Conclusion	97
	Bibliography	97
10	**Interlude V: Grief and Humor**	**99**
10.1	Grief is not a Disease	100
10.2	Stages of Grief	100
10.3	Numbness and Stupor:	101
10.4	Sadness and Longing:	101
10.5	Disorganisation, Searching and Separation	102
10.6	New Orientation and Recovery	102
10.7	Laughing Tears: Grief and Humor	103
10.8	Humor as a Coping Strategy	103
10.9	Humor and Cynicism	104
	Further Reading	105
11	**Carl Gustav Jung (1875–1961): Anticipation of the Coming Adventure**	**107**
11.1	Personality No. 1 and No. 2	109
11.2	Mother	110
11.3	Father	110
11.4	Family	110
11.5	Faints	111
11.6	High School	111

11.7	Studies	111
11.8	Burghölzli	112
11.9	Dissertation	112
11.10	Starting a Family	113
11.11	Jung's Relationship with Freud	113
11.12	Points of Contention	114
11.13	Analytical Psychology	115
11.14	The Scandalous Affair: Sabina Spielrein	115
11.15	Toni Wolff	116
11.16	Private Practice and Travels	116
11.17	The Reputation Rises	116
11.18	National Socialism	116
11.19	Honesty and Humility	117
11.20	Near-Death Experiences	118
11.21	Suffering Success	118
11.22	Death of the Wife	119
11.23	Preparations for Dying	120
11.24	Initial Dreams	120
11.25	Death Wedding Procession	121
11.26	Saying Goodbye	121
11.27	"How wonderful …"	122
11.28	Hour of Death	122
11.29	Synchronicity and Reincarnation	122
11.30	Funeral	123
11.31	Conclusion	124
	Bibliography	124

12 Interlude VI: Finiteness—Lifetime—Dying Time (Small Exercises) — 125

12.1	The Temporal Questions	126
12.2	How Do I Want to Die?	126
12.3	And After?	127
	Further Reading	127

13 Karlfried Graf Dürckheim (1896–1988): Endured Pain During Conscious Transition — 129

13.1	First Experience with Death	131
13.2	Military Service in the 1st World War	131
13.3	Studies	132
13.4	Religion and Mysticism	132
13.5	University of Leipzig	132

13.6	Nazi Era	133
13.7	Japan and Zen	133
13.8	Todtmoos-Rütte	134
13.9	Initiatic Therapy	134
13.10	Rütte Impulse	136
13.11	Appreciation	136
13.12	Limitations	137
13.13	The Door Opens Inward	137
13.14	Daily Routine	138
13.15	In the Face of Death	138
13.16	Hour of Death	139
13.17	Conclusion	139
	Further Reading	140

14 Interlude VII: Images of Humans and Therapy Goals in Psychotherapy — 141
Further Reading — 144

15 Nossrat Peseschkian (1933–2010): Death in Sleep — 145

15.1	Origin and Extended Family	147
15.2	Kashan	147
15.3	Mother	147
15.4	Baha'i	148
15.5	School Time	149
15.6	Father	149
15.7	Music and Literature	150
15.8	Medicine	150
15.9	Wanderer between Two Worlds	151
15.10	German Language—difficult Language	151
15.11	Studies	152
15.12	Bridge Builder	152
15.13	From Body to Psyche	153
15.14	Private Practice	153
15.15	Myth Therapy and Differentiation Analysis	154
15.16	Positive Psychotherapy	154
15.17	Positum	155
15.18	Publications	156
15.19	Balance Model: Four Areas of Life	157
15.20	The Three Stages of Interaction	159
15.21	The Five-Step Treatment Strategy:	160
15.22	Use of Stories, Aphorisms, Jokes	162

15.23	The Other View of Symptoms	163
15.24	Personal Contact	164
15.25	Active Until the Last Moment	165
15.26	Funeral	166
15.27	Further Development	166
15.28	Conclusion	167
Bibliography		167

16 Epilogue: Live Your Dying   169
Further Reading   173

About the Author

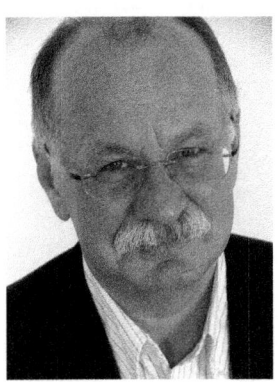

Werner Gross, Graduate Psychologist, Psychotherapist, Supervisor and Coach, Organizational and Business Consultant. He runs a psychological practice in Gelnhausen (Germany) and is lecturer for psychology at various universities and training institutes for psychotherapists.

1

Sigmund Freud (1856–1939): The Morphine-Dulled Pain of Dying

Contents

1.1	Childhood and Youth	3
1.2	Studies	4
1.3	Josef Breuer	4
1.4	Martha Bernays—Starting a Family	5
1.5	Cocaine	5
1.6	Charcot and Hypnosis	6
1.7	From Physiology to Psychology	6
1.8	Cathartic Method	7
1.9	Wilhelm Fließ	7
1.10	Free Association and Couch	7
1.11	Psychoanalysis	8
1.12	Sexuality	8
1.13	Self-analysis: Where Id was, Ego shall be	8
1.14	Psychoanalytic Movement	9
1.15	Marriage and Family	9
1.16	Physical Constitution and Diseases	9
1.17	Libido and Destrudo	10
1.18	The Destruction of the Life's Work	11
1.19	Exile in London	12
1.20	Euthanasia Morphine	12
1.21	Sapere aude	13
1.22	The Third Great Humiliation of Humanity	13
1.23	Conclusion	14
Further Reading		14

© The Author(s), under exclusive license to Springer-Verlag GmbH, DE, part of Springer Nature 2024
W. Gross, *As One Lives, So One Dies*, https://doi.org/10.1007/978-3-662-70061-7_1

> This chapter is about the portrayal of the life of Sigmund Freud, that is, how the stern, serious father of psychoanalysis lived, how he died, and how the cool analyst, who wanted to turn the Id into the Ego, did not want to simply face death unconsciously. It revolves around his tenacious struggle with "the monster", the oral prosthesis. He fights against his cancer and yet persists in his excessive cigar consumption, even though it is closely linked to his terminal illness. In this 16-year-long battle, he develops his death drive theory ("Destrudo") and in the end, has his family doctor inject him with an overdose of morphine.

Whoever constantly understands what he is doing, remains below his level. (Martin Walser)

> **Overview**
> Imagine you had spent many years of your life working and fighting for your idea, your worldview and method. You would have invested all your energy and vigor, your "brainpower" and your "heart and soul" into it. You would have always stood up for this idea, always believed that this idea—even if you would only experience it in its early stages during your lifetime—would bring about a drastic change in the image of mankind.
>
> On the one hand, your theory would have found its way into everyday language and the vocabulary of many languages. And on the other hand—besides the undeniable successes of your work—you would have experienced hostility from colleagues and the general public, endured envy, jealousy, ridicule, and even contempt. You would have put your marriage, your family, your children on the back burner for life and discarded friendships for it. And now—at the end of your life—your idea would be "murdered"—just like that and without a chance to defend yourself. You would have had to flee to another country. Your relatives would be exposed to persecution and this in a situation where you would have had to endure severe pain and physical limitations for years. And now injustice simply takes away everything you have suffered, loved, and lived for. Can you imagine how tired you would be? Perhaps even tired of life? This is probably how Sigmund Freud felt at the end of his life.

"The cancer ate its way through the cheeks to the outside, and with it, the risk of sepsis increased," describes his most important biographer, Ernest Jones, the last days of Sigmund Freud. Since he had to flee Vienna from the Nazis, he has been living in London for over a year and although he still treats patients there, he is now in a state of extreme exhaustion. He must have felt indescribably miserable during this time.

On September 19, 1939, Ernest Jones visits Freud one last time to say his final goodbye. As Freud dozes off exhausted, he only briefly opens his eyes when he recognizes Jones, raises his hand in greeting, and lets it fall again—before he falls back asleep—with a resigned gesture. It says: It's over. Words are no longer necessary. Everything has been said. "Whereof one cannot speak, thereof one must be silent," echoing this sentence by Ludwig Wittgenstein, only silence remains.

According to statements by Freud's family doctor Max Schur, Freud called him on September 21. Freud begins softly: "Dear Schur, you probably remember our first conversation. You promised me then to help me when I can't go on. This is now just torture and makes no sense anymore."

When Schur squeezes Freud's hand and tells him that he has not forgotten his promise and will keep it, Freud sighs with relief, holds Schur's hand for a moment longer and says: "Thank you."

He then adds: "Please tell Anna about our conversation."

There is little self-pity, only reality.—Not only for Schur an impressive and unforgettable scene.

The following day, on September 22, Schur gives Freud a third of a grain of morphine. For someone who is so exhausted and unfamiliar with opiates, this small dose is enough. He sighs with relief and sinks—obviously at the end of his strength—into a peaceful sleep.

The next day, September 23, 1939, around 3 a.m., he dies.

Ernest Jones, Freud's most important biographer writes: "His long and arduous life is over and all suffering is past. Freud dies as he lived—as a realist."

Jones thus describes the death of the man who, with the development of psychoanalysis, influenced the world and human image of the 20th century like hardly any other person.

Terms that we use today as a matter of course, such as "unconscious", "sublimation", "slip of the tongue", "dream interpretation", "Oedipus complex", "defense mechanisms", "libido", "superego" can be traced back to Freud and psychoanalysis.

1.1 Childhood and Youth

Sigismund Freud was born on May 6, 1856, in the small Moravian town of Freiberg, the son of the 41-year-old Jewish cloth merchant Jacob Freud and his wife Amalia, who was 20 years younger. From his father's first marriage, there are the two much older half-brothers Emanuel and Philip.

Philip, who is 20 years old, already has a one-year-old son who becomes Sigismund's favorite playmate. Thus, Sigismund is in the curious situation of being born as an uncle. He is the first son of his then 21-year-old mother and probably also her favorite. In 1910 he writes:

"If one has been the undisputed favorite of the mother, one retains for life that feeling of conquest, that confidence of success, which often indeed brings success."

Seven more siblings are born in the following years. Soon after the birth of Sigismund, the father runs into business difficulties and the family decides to leave Freiberg when the son is 3 years old, first moving to Saxony, then settling in Vienna in 1860. Throughout his childhood, the family lives in rather meager circumstances. Nevertheless, the father sends his son to high school at the age of 9, a year earlier than usual.

Freud is a top student for long stretches of his school time and passes the Matura, the Austrian high school graduation, with distinction ("summa cum laude"). He is very well-read and reads texts in several languages. Even then, he is congratulated on his linguistic talent and his good German style.

1.2 Studies

At the age of 17, Freud goes to university in Vienna and begins to study medicine, after some experimentation with other subjects. In a note about his life, he writes that from his early years he was "unaware of any need to help suffering people." Rather, in his youth, the need to understand something of the mysteries of the world and perhaps to contribute something to their solution was overwhelming.

Freud studies medicine for 15 semesters, which he pursues "quite negligently". First, he dissects river eels and studies the nervous system of crustaceans. Until it becomes clear to him that he is primarily interested in humans. The biological origin of mental processes and neurology is his topic during this time.

1.3 Josef Breuer

In 1878, Freud is now 22 years old, when he changes his first name from Sigismund to Sigmund. A close friendship develops with the 14 years older Viennese doctor and scientist Josef Breuer even before his doctoral examination. Breuer becomes Freud's mentor and supports him not only emotionally, but also materially through generous loans.

In 1881, he (belatedly) passes the final exams and is eventually promoted to doctor.

However, general medicine bores him and Freud decides to stop his quite fruitful research work and end his scientific career—also because his chances of getting a free professorship are slim. His next goal is to practice as a doctor. He also writes that he had no particular preference for the position and activity of a doctor.

In his *self-portrayal*, he says that the turning point came in 1882 when his "highly revered teacher" Breuer corrected the generous recklessness of his father by urgently warning him to give up the theoretical career. Financial reasons probably also influenced him, as he wants to start a family and that requires fiscal security.

1.4 Martha Bernays—Starting a Family

The new career path that Freud now embarks on is primarily determined by the fact that he secretly gets engaged to Martha Bernays in June 1882 and from now on strives to create the material basis for his marriage to her. Martha Bernays comes from a Jewish intellectual family. His letters to Martha during their engagement are still full of passions, fears, unjustified jealousies, and uncertainties. So he writes to Martha in the summer of 1884:

"Woe, little princess, when I come. I will kiss you all red and feed you very thick, and if you are naughty, you will see who is stronger, a little gentle girl who doesn't eat, or a big wild man who has cocaine in his body."

In 1886, he marries Martha Bernays and later has 6 children with her. From then on, Freud's external life is constant. His family life is in calm waters and leaves him enough time for his practice and almost his studies. Until he has to flee the Nazis to London, he lives almost 50 years in the same apartment in Vienna.

1.5 Cocaine

But Freud also remains faithful to research alongside his practice. In particular, cocaine and its properties fascinate him during this time. In the following years, he deals—both scientifically and in self-experiments—with the properties of cocaine, the effects of which were not yet known at that time.

He writes a monograph titled *On Coca*, which makes him known in professional circles.

Critics of Freud claim (sometimes to this day) that he was addicted to cocaine for long stretches of his life.

1.6 Charcot and Hypnosis

But a completely different topic is increasingly becoming the focus of his interest: Hypnosis.

He receives a scholarship for a study trip to Paris to Jean Martin Charcot, who runs the Parisian neurological-psychiatric institution Salpetrière and experiments there with hypnosis—especially on hysterical patients.

The Salpetrière is something like the Mecca of neurologists at this time and Charcot is the prophet.

Freud greatly admires Charcot, as he dignifiedly walks through the old-fashioned halls of this hospital and names a whole series of nervous diseases "just like Adam once named the creatures of creation" (Jones 1984).

For Freud, Charcot is a significant personality: strong and powerful, yet kind, benevolent, and witty.

After Charcot's death in 1893, Freud writes of "the magic that emanated from his appearance and voice, the gracious openness" … Freud admires the willingness with which he makes everything available to his students, and the loyalty he maintains to them throughout life.

For him, Charcot as a teacher is captivating. And each of his lectures was a small work of art in structure and organization, perfect and so compelling that one had to think about the spoken word all day.

Certainly, Freud is very much shaped by the person of Charcot—especially since he works almost 5 months in the Salpetrière.

1.7 From Physiology to Psychology

His work takes—after returning to Vienna—a radical turn: He takes the decisive step from physiology and neurology to psychology and psychiatry.

When Freud worked in Paris, Charcot—as mentioned—was interested in hypnosis and especially the treatment of hysteria. In the medical world, both were considered unprofessional and offensive at the time, and in a lecture to the Viennese medical profession about Charcot's hysteria doctrine, he mainly encounters rejection.

He experiments in his practice with the "electrification method" for treating "nervous disorders", but is very dissatisfied with it and almost simultaneously begins to work with hypnosis.

He translates a book from French about hypnosis and works with his old friend Josef Breuer, who performs the "cathartic method" with hysterical patients.

1.8 Cathartic Method

The assumption of this cathartic Method is that hysteria is the product of a psychological injury, a trauma, that the patients have forgotten.

The treatment consists of putting the patients into a hypnotic trance and then suggesting to them to remember the forgotten trauma with the associated feelings. This often leads to crying or screaming fits and the patients often feel relieved afterwards. However, the state rarely lasts long and only in individual cases does this treatment lead to a complete cure.

Therefore, Freud soon begins to change the therapy procedure—and also the theoretical explanatory model on which it is based. This new method and his formulation of the hypothesis of "traumatic seduction" leads to an open break with his long-time friend and mentor Josef Breuer.

1.9 Wilhelm Fließ

In 1887, Freud meets the Berlin ENT doctor Wilhelm Fließ at an evening party hosted by Breuer. Since he also attended Freud's lectures, they also find the scientific basis for a collaboration. Fließ, who is 2 years younger than Freud and very imaginative, comes from a Sephardic Jewish family and becomes Freud's "alter ego", his intimate friend, with whom he exchanges exactly 284 letters from 1887 to 1902.

Fließ becomes for him a "resonator" and "thought amplifier". They send each other their scientific works, meet at regular intervals and explain their projects and thoughts to each other. The discussions about Fließ's theories ("periodicity theory" and "nasal reflex neurosis") and the development of Freudian psychoanalysis are productive for almost 15 years, until there is a dispute about whether a genuinely psychological causation must always be in the foreground in the development of neuroses. This leads to an irreconcilable disagreement.

1.10 Free Association and Couch

Freud no longer puts his patients into a hypnotic trance during his "talking cure", but lets them in their normal state of consciousness. This then develops over the years into the psychoanalytic technique of "free association", to which the patients are encouraged in a certain setting in therapy: On the now legendary "couch" the patient lies, while the analyst sits behind him at his head end.

1.11 Psychoanalysis

The year is 1896 when the word "Psychoanalysis" is used for the first time. Freud publishes a sensational theory the same year: Every hysteria, he concludes from the reports of his patients, has its cause in a sexual trauma in early childhood. This can involve rapes or incestuous experiences.

His lectures at the university about the sexual causes of hysteria lead to great excitement among his colleagues and to a scandal. He is rejected and laughed at. Thus, he gradually drifts into an almost 6-year isolation at the university.

1.12 Sexuality

Although sexuality plays a central role in Freud's theory of man, he himself claims—also because of his early and close bond with his wife Martha—to have enjoyed little of sexual freedom. In a letter to James Putnam, he wrote in 1915:

"I advocate a much freer sexual life, although I myself have practiced very little of such freedom."

And he believes that unexpressed (sexual) feelings will never die. In his opinion, they are buried alive and later emerge in an ugly way. Unless they are transformed ("sublimation").

Critics not particularly fond of psychoanalysis therefore also believe that the entire psychoanalysis is nothing more than the processing of Freud's personal problems with his sexuality.

1.13 Self-analysis: Where Id was, Ego shall be

In the summer of 1897, Freud begins his self-analysis. He writes to a friend: "The main patient who occupies me is myself."

From this self-analysis significant parts flow into his important books *The Interpretation of Dreams* and *The Psychopathology of Everyday Life*, which appear around the turn of the century. Only slowly does the isolation in which Freud has long found himself dissolve.

1.14 Psychoanalytic Movement

From 1902, Sigmund Freud meets weekly with students, including Alfred Adler, Wilhelm Stekel, Otto Rank, and later C. G. Jung, for the so-called psychological Wednesday society. From 1908, this became the "Vienna Psychoanalytic Association"—the nucleus of the "International Psychoanalytic Association" founded in 1910.

He publishes further significant works such as *Three Essays on the Theory of Sexuality* or *The Joke and Its Relation to the Unconscious*. The first psychoanalytic congresses are held, the first psychoanalytic journal is published.

Slowly over the next few years, the psychoanalytic movement grows, initially exclusively in Vienna, later also in Berlin and Zurich, where C. G. Jung, who is Freud's student from 1906–1912, and works at a psychiatric clinic in Switzerland, the "Burghölzli" (more on this see Chap. 11).

Psychoanalysis is increasingly stepping into the public spotlight. It is being talked about in many intellectual circles—and jokes are being made about it.

Psychoanalysis is not only applied to individual mental life, but Freud also includes societal issues in *Group Psychology and the Analysis of the Ego* and in *Beyond the Pleasure Principle*.

1.15 Marriage and Family

In stark contrast to the professional excitement is the domestic situation: He has been married to Martha Bernays since 1886 and has 6 children. The youngest, Anna, will be the only one to continue her father's work. His private life is characterized by continuity and balance. From 1891–1938 he lives and practices in the same house at Berggasse 19 in Vienna, until he has to flee the Nazis to London.

1.16 Physical Constitution and Diseases

Freud's end does not come unexpectedly, it is the result of a long history of illness. Although in his younger years Freud certifies himself a strong constitution in a letter to his future wife Martha. Throughout his life, however, he suffers from minor and major illnesses:

A mild form of typhus in 1882, a smallpox infection in 1885—albeit without scars, rheumatic diseases, heart complaints, functional gastrointestinal disorders, but above all diseases of the nose-mouth-throat area.

Finally: Freud is a heavy smoker all his life. He does not want and cannot give up cigar smoking even when he is diagnosed with oral cancer at the age of 67 in 1923.

He has to undergo a total of 33 operations in the oral cavity area from 1923 until his death in 1939. He almost bled to death the night after the first operation, if not for a "dwarf cretin" who shared the room with him and got help.

The surgeon has decided to remove the diseased tissue as radically as possible. Both the hard palate and parts of the soft palate fall victim to the scalpel, so that the partition between the oral and nasal cavities disappears.

The consequences for Freud—besides the fear of bleeding—are far-reaching and terrible. He has to wear a prosthesis that hinders him so much when eating that he prefers to eat alone. The severity of the change is also shown by the fact that the psychoanalyst has to pry open his dentures with a clothespin to be able to push his beloved cigar between his teeth. In addition, the prosthesis irritates the oral mucosa and often causes secondary diseases, inflammations, and ulcers.

Speaking is also difficult for him. His pronunciation becomes slurred, unclear-nasal and he is sometimes barely understandable. Public speeches are from then on the exception—which also means that he has to refrain from attending the psychoanalytic congresses and giving speeches there.

1.17 Libido and Destrudo

It is probably no coincidence that Freud developed the concept of a death drive "Destrudo" parallel to the life drive "Libido" during this time.

In 1931, 8 years after the initial diagnosis, a catastrophic turn of events occurs: a malignant tumor robs Freud of any hope for a final cure.

From then on at the latest, Freud must come to terms with the fact that he inevitably carries the disease to death within him. The carcinoma leaves no room for self-deception anymore. It is like a silent witness, reminding of the secret progress of death. In 1933, he believes that the *New Lectures on Psychoanalysis*, which he has just finished, will be his last work. Already in July 1936, another malignant tumor has to be removed. Radiation therapy is initiated and the discomfort caused by the radiation adds to the pain of the disease—bleeding in the mouth, headaches, dizziness. In addition, there is the constant struggle with the "monster", the prosthesis. Because of the pain, he finds it difficult to sleep. He loses weight—also because of the discomfort when eating—extremely, can only speak with difficulty and feels weak and miserable. Because of the great pain after chronic insomnia, his doctors advise him to take painkillers and sedatives. His answer:

"I would rather think in agony than not be able to think clearly."

This sounds heroic and pathetic, but it is only the desire not to go unconsciously towards death. But the sentence of Socrates also applies:

"Better to be an unhappy philosopher than a happy pig."

The fact that death becomes such a topic for Freud during this time is also evident in the development of the death drive—"Destrudo".

Just as "Libido" is to be understood as the urge and desire for life (and is associated with the Greek god "Eros"), "Destrudo" is to be understood as the manifestation of the destructive, of death (and expression of "Thanatos" the god of death). And although Freud had already found the idea of Destrudo as a precursor through the horrors of the 1st World War, he only really developed the concept in the 1920s, when the cancer in him was in full bloom. This concept of "Destrudo" as the opposite term to "Libido" is still controversial in psychoanalysis today.

1.18 The Destruction of the Life's Work

Parallel to Freud's decline, the threatening political situation in Germany unfolds: The Nazis' are in power, the persecution of Jews begins. His life's work is threatened and gradually destroyed. His books are burned with the saying:

"Against the soul-destroying overestimation of sexual life and for the nobility of the human soul—I consign to the flames the writings of a certain Sigmund Freud."

Freud sarcastically comments:

"What progress we are making: In the Middle Ages they would have burned me, nowadays they are content to burn my books."

Although he is still appointed a member of the "Royal Society" in Great Britain in 1936, resignation has now gained the upper hand. In a letter to Arnold Zweig, he writes:

"One should not be deceived that this time rejects me and what I had to give, and is not willing to be disturbed in its judgment by shouts. Probably my time will still come, but—for now it is over."

The only thing left for him is writing. It is as a refuge, the possibility to escape resignation, and it is his old passion.

It is also interesting that he confesses:

"I am not a man of science at all, not an observer, not an experimenter, not a thinker. I am a conquistador talent, an adventurer with the curiosity, the boldness, and the tenacity of such."

He finishes *Moses and Monotheism* and some smaller writings, of which the most significant *Analysis Terminable and Interminable* becomes of fundamental importance for psychoanalysis.

Wherever the Nazis arrive, Freud's work is destroyed. The psychoanalytic institutes are closed, the assets confiscated, the psychoanalysts driven into emigration.

By 1939—in Freud's year of death—there is no longer a psychoanalytic institute on the European mainland.

1.19 Exile in London

When the Nazis also take power in Austria in 1938 and the Gestapo interrogates Freud's son daily, later also his favorite daughter Anna, and threatens him and his family with the concentration camp, he decides to go into exile in London.

As a last harassment (and as a condition for the actual departure to England), he should sign a form of the Gestapo, which says:

"I gladly confirm that until today, June 4, 1938, no harassment of my person or my housemates has occurred. Authorities and party officials have always treated me and my housemates with consideration." It is rumored that Freud added in handwriting: "I can highly recommend the Gestapo to everyone."

With great difficulty, he finally arrives—eyed by the sympathy of the world press—via Paris in London. London welcomes him with public attention. The Freuds "drown in flowers". At the end of Regent's Park, in the north of London, Freud moves into his last apartment, where he still receives patients.

1.20 Euthanasia Morphine

On September 21, 1939, he asks his family doctor Max Schur for help. From now on, everything is just torture, he says. The next day, Schur gives him a third of a grain of morphine. On September 23, at 3 a.m., Sigmund Freud dies without ever waking up again.

He dies in pain, but almost silently. Throughout his life, he was rational and not very emotional. He decides for himself about dying when the disease leaves him no more strength to work.

1.21 Sapere aude

It is hard to imagine Freud in tears, lost in fits of rage, or running amok in despair. Emotional explosions must have been alien to him. Freud died in pain, but quietly.

He seems to have slowly coagulated or silted up. What he says or writes is rational, thoughtful, and if emotional, then very maturely emotional throughout his life.—And this, even though he dealt with feelings—especially in childhood. This is how his work—psychoanalysis—is, and this is how he died.

"Sapere aude" (dare to know) was his credo!

The psychoanalyst Johannes Cremerius writes that Freud died as he lived. For him, Freud is a unity of work, life, and death. Even when Freud makes the decision that there is no longer any point in living because the disease has consumed all his strength, he dies in freedom by opening the door to death.

1.22 The Third Great Humiliation of Humanity

Freud was nominated for the Nobel Prize several times—both for medicine and for literature. He did not receive it, although he is considered one of the most important thinkers of the 20th century. After all, Sigmund Freud is the person who inflicted the third great humiliation on human narcissism:

The first humiliation goes back to **Copernicus**, who proved that it is not the sun that revolves around the earth, but the earth that revolves around the sun. Thus, the earth is not the center of the universe. A severe insult to human-centered fantasies of grandeur, that the earth as a human home is the navel of the cosmos—as medieval Christianity always invoked, proclaimed, and defended.

The second humiliation is inflicted on humanity by Charles **Darwin**, who saw humans as the result of evolution (not as a unique and unchangeable crown of creation) and thus dethroned humans.

Freud, with the development of psychoanalysis, proved that man is not even "master in his own house". He is all too often at the mercy of his unconscious, his drives, and can only control himself consciously and voluntarily to a limited extent. Perhaps this third humiliation of humanity is the most massive of all …

1.23 Conclusion

Freud, the strict, serious father of psychoanalysis, the realist, the cool analyst, who wanted to turn the "Id" into "Ego", does not want to face death unconsciously. The tough fight against "the monster", against the mouth prosthesis, and against cancer corresponds in a certain sense to a continuity with which he, for example, clings to his excessive cigar consumption, like a beloved symptom, even though it is closely related to his fatal illness. This 16-year-long fight against cancer, during which "Destrudo", his death drive theory, emerges, ends with a very purposefully used dose of morphine, which—almost like suicide—leads to death.

Further Reading

Cremerius, Johannes: Sigmund Freud in „Letzte Tage" Eds. Von H. J. Schultz, Stuttgart 1983 (Kreuz)
Freud, Sigmund: Studienausgabe, Vol. 1–10, Frankfurt/M. 1969, (S. Fischer)
Fromm, Erich: Sigmund Freud, Berlin 1981 (Ullstein)
Gidal, Tim: Die Freudianer, München 1990 (Verlag internat. Psychoanalyse)
Jones, Ernest: Sigmund Freud, Leben und Werk, Bd. 1–3, München 1984 (dtv)
Mannoni, Octave: Freud – Reinbek bei Hamburg, 1971 (rororo-Monographien)
Schur, Max: Sigmund Freud, Leben und Sterben, Frankfurt/M. 1979 (Suhrkamp)
Sulloway, Frank J.: Freud – Biologe der Seele. Jenseits der psychoanalytischen Legende, Köln-Lövenich 1982 (Edition Maschke)

2

Interlude I: On Aging

Contents

2.1 Wisdom in Old Age—Senility—Stubbornness in Old Age. 16
2.2 Three Types of Age 17
2.3 Review 17
Further Reading 18

> This is about the various aspects of age: chronological, biological, and psychological age. It's about wisdom in old age, senility, and stubbornness in old age, and what one can do to develop the right attitude to deal with aging appropriately.

Everyone wants to become it—no one wants to be it: old.

"Growing old is not for the faint-hearted," is a quote attributed to one of the early Hollywood sex symbols, actress Mae West. The late Edgar Wallace detective and television presenter Joachim Fuchsberger even made it a book title in 2014.

And indeed: Almost everyone wishes for a long life, but preferably in good health, with as few restrictions as possible, and ideally, filled with intense life events and wisdom: "I am life that wants to live, in the midst of life that wants to live," Albert Schweitzer is said to have stated.

In reality, it is not so easy to age with dignity, to deal appropriately with the limitations and infirmities—the back problems, the sleep disorders, the hearing and vision difficulties, the delayed thought processes, the movement restrictions, and the other age-related ailments.

And this, of course, also applies to psychotherapists—they too age and feel where it begins to end and where it ends to begin. They too must learn to counteract the entropy, the decay process of life. How differently the great psychotherapists presented here have done this—each in his own way—can be read in the individual chapters.

2.1 Wisdom in Old Age—Senility—Stubbornness in Old Age

But dealing with aging affects us all—we must learn to deal appropriately with our aging processes.

Evil people claim that in old age one can only—more or less consciously—choose between: wisdom in old age, senility and stubbornness in old age—albeit in different degrees and mixtures. However, there is indeed a much broader choice:

Some become active and try to counteract the aging process by activating the body. According to the motto: "Forever young—Age, you won't get me down: I won't let myself go, I'll go myself." Self-control and self-discipline is their motto. In extreme cases, they participate in marathons, or even torture themselves in the Ironman Triathlon. "He who always does what he can already do, remains always what he already is," said Henry Ford. "When was the last time you did something for the first time?"

Others try to realize their unfulfilled dreams, buy a Harley Davidson or a convertible sports coupe, and try to enjoy as much as possible.

Some desperately search for the 3rd spring, have fat suctioned off here and wrinkles botoxed away there, or chase after the latest fashion trends.

Still others humbly surrender to their fate or ironize their desires:

"Clear up top and tight down below, dear God, that's all I want," goes a bon mot. Everyone has their individual pattern to deal with the tender indifference of life. As long as one fights, nothing is lost.

One thing is certain—the proportion of late-adolescent pensioners is increasing, all of whom are trying to catch up on what they believe they have missed in their lives.

2.2 Three Types of Age

Basically, one can distinguish three types of age:

- The **calendar** age. There is nothing to change about it, because every day has 24 h, every hour has 60 minutes, and every minute has 60 seconds. This is objective time. The question is at most what one uses the time for, whether one wastes it or lets the brain run on "autopilot" and indulges in a more or less meaningful routine, or whether one uses the time consciously.
- The **biological** age is related to how well our organs, our skeletal structure, our joints, and our senses are. This is certainly partly determined by our genetics, our constitution, but also our lifestyle. What patterns have you developed over the years—how long-term healthy are they? And for which sins do you pay in later age?
- The **psychological** age is the most flexible: "You are as young as you feel." On a psychological level, it shows that age is also a question of attitude. Do I still give my life a chance? What am I looking forward to when I get up in the morning? When was the last time I did something for the first time? Goals could be: stay open to new experiences. Having a goal, a project, an idea to realize, keeps you young. As long as you remain curious, you are young—at least in your head. *With maturity, you get younger and younger* is a booklet subtitled by Hermann Hesse …

Of course, these three aspects of age are interconnected, but they are not identical. It is therefore useful to differentiate them because they can be influenced differently by will: You can't change the **calendar** age at all. The **biological** age can only be influenced in the long term through a changed lifestyle, while the **psychological** age can very well be influenced (e.g., through psychotherapy) by a changed inner attitude—sometimes even dramatically. You can say: The glass is already half empty or it is still half full. Both perspectives are realistic—but it makes a big difference in terms of experience: You may not be able to give life more days,—but you can give more life to the days.

2.3 Review

Growing old is like mountain climbing. The higher you climb, the more your strength fades, but the further you see. (Ingmar Bergman)

As at the end of a long mountain hike, it is definitely worthwhile to take a look at the past life path: What were the grand peaks that one has climbed in one's life—after the efforts of the ascent? What were the deep valleys? What were the painstakingly traversed plains, what were the falls and injuries, the misdirections and dead ends …?

But also, what was good, where was the effort worthwhile, at which crossroads did one hesitate and doubt—and then (more or less) consciously continued on one's life path. Whatever happened to you and whatever you did—the past cannot be changed. What has happened has happened—but one can learn from it for the remaining lifetime: What do I want to keep in the time remaining to me—and what to change?

"Give every day the chance to be the best of your life," Mark Twain once wrote. One could add: no matter how old you are.

If you have a hard time with it, sometimes the support of a psychotherapist or a coach can help.

Don't be upset that it's over. Be glad that it was and that you experienced it.

The basic question is—have I just gotten old or have I understood something? Have I just (more or less cleverly) gotten through life or have I become smart—or even a little wise?

Further Reading

Hercher, Frank: Was heißt hier „altes Eisen"? Wiesbaden 1989 (Hercher)
Kusch, Rita: Schatztruhe für die Seniorenarbeit, Gütersloh 2015 (Gütersloher Verlagshaus)
Likar, Rudolf et al.: Lebensqualität im Alter, Wien 2005 (Springer)
Pretat, Jane R.: Dem Alter entgegenreifen, Zürich 1996 (Walter)
Schnack, Gerd + Kirsten, Rauhe, Hermann: Jung bleiben kann man lernen, München 2002 (Kösel)
VELKD (Vereinigte Evangelisch-Lutherische Kirche Deutschlands): Lust und Last der späten Jahre, Gütersloh 2016 (Gütersloher Verlagshaus)
Willen, Günther: Wer das liest, lebt länger, Bern 2003 (Scherz)

3

Alfred Adler (1870–1937): Sudden Death During a Walk

Contents

3.1	Childhood and First Illnesses	21
3.2	Family Situation	22
3.3	School, Studies, and Start of Career	23
3.4	Starting a Family	23
3.5	Freud—Adler	24
3.6	Setting Variables	24
3.7	Separation	25
3.8	Individual Psychology	25
3.9	Compensation Ability	26
3.10	Unconscious Life Plan	27
3.11	Community Feeling and Life Goal	27
3.12	Activities	27
3.13	Educational Counseling Centers and Children's Clinics	28
3.14	Adler's Image of Humanity	28
3.15	Educational Ideas in "Red Vienna"	29
3.16	Publications and Lecture Tours	30
3.17	Relocation to the USA	30
3.18	Last Days	31
3.19	Cremation and Honorary Grave in Vienna	32
3.20	The Social Genius	32
3.21	Conclusion	32
Bibliography		33

> **Trailer**
>
> This chapter is about the life and death of Alfred Adler—and its connection to the development of his method, individual psychology.
>
> Adler is the rather life-loving, socially committed, warm-hearted helper type and the representative of an "optimistic psychology", in whose theory death does not play a central role. As he travels almost hectically through the USA and Europe to spread his individual psychology, he succumbs—completely unexpectedly—and without a long struggle to death, to a heart attack.

The greatest danger in life is that one becomes too cautious. (Alfred Adler)

> **Overview**
>
> Some people manage to maintain certain basic patterns in their lives, more or less consciously. For example, first-borns may grow up with the feeling of having the natural right to always and everywhere be in the front row (or even have to be).
>
> For second-borns, the exact opposite may be the case, so they often have the feeling of being at the back, in second place—which not everyone likes. If then the own narcissistic desire for attention and admiration from others develops, this can lead to an inner conflict that sooner or later seeps out through the buttonholes and also shows in dealing with other people.
>
> Because from this "inferiority complex" and the old struggle with the first-born, something like a life theme can later develop, which is more or less (un)consciously re-enacted in all possible relationships later in life—be it in the group with peers and colleagues or with superiors or bosses:
>
> Often it is about the topic of rivalry—with someone who is admired on the one hand and despised on the other, but whose role and position one would like to have. Symbolically one could say: to admire someone on one's knees and despise or fight them.
>
> This rivalry can show itself—more or less openly. It is then about the struggle of who is the better one.
>
> Perhaps this also shows up in the relationship between Alfred Adler and Sigmund Freud.

"For a Jewish boy from a Viennese suburb, a death in Aberdeen is in itself an outrageous career and proof of how far he has come. … Indeed, the world has richly rewarded him for opposing psychoanalysis."

This quote does not come from the pen of a stubborn Freud-hater—it is not about Sigmund Freud at all—but this is how maliciously Freud himself wrote about one of his—according to his own account—most talented students in a letter to Arnold Zweig:

Alfred Adler is meant, who worked closely with Freud from 1902–1911, but later opposed Freud's emphasis on sexuality and the drive life. For Adler, who broke away from Freud's psychoanalysis in 1911 and founded "Individual Psychology", other terms are in the foreground:

Organ inferiority and Inferiority complex, the will to power, community feeling and the goal orientation of human life.

As with Freud, it can also be shown with Adler how much the therapeutic concept that a person develops is connected with his personal history and is first and foremost an attempt to understand himself and the world and to order it using a theoretical framework.

Let's take the term "organ inferiority" or more popularly the "inferiority complex". It is closely linked to the person Alfred Adler and his personal biography.

3.1 Childhood and First Illnesses

Alfred Adler was born on February 7, 1870, in a suburb of Vienna as the second-born son of a total of 7 children of the wealthy grain merchant Leopold Adler and his wife Pauline.

In individual psychology, Adler later points out that second-born children often develop into the "ambitious type" by training from childhood to be on par with the older child. Thus, Alfred Adler initially emulates his 2-year-old older brother in childhood, who later becomes a successful businessman, while Alfred is successful in a completely different field.

Here we also find a close connection with the term "Will to Power"—a rivalry that he eventually also carries out with Freud. Freud and his older brother, by the way, both have the same first name: Sigmund …

Something else influences Adler's view of the world much more. Adler suffers from rickets and a laryngeal spasm in his childhood, which mainly occurs when crying—in individual psychological terms, a real "Organ Inferiority". Adler writes: "From my youth history, I remember several events in which death seemed close to me." Adler reports that he had a laryngeal spasm quite often due to rickets—and difficulty moving… "where the closure of the glottis occurs during crying, so that a state of breathlessness and voicelessness interrupts the crying until the spasm is resolved and the crying continues. The state of breathlessness that occurs is extremely unpleasant, as I know from my memory: I must have been not yet three years old…" (Adler 1986, p. 120).

Elsewhere he formulates further that one day, shortly after such a wheezing attack, he had thoughts "how I, since no remedy had worked so far, could eliminate this annoying suffering… I decided to stop crying altogether, and as soon as I felt the first urge to cry, I gave myself a jerk, stopped crying, and the wheezing disappeared. I had found a remedy for the suffering, perhaps also for the fear of death." (Adler 1986, p. 120).

The will to survive of the young Alfred is even more strongly shaped by another experience, which ultimately also tips the balance for the choice of the later medical profession:

"At the age of five, I fell ill with pneumonia and was given up by the doctor. A second doctor suggested a treatment, and I was healthy in a few days. In the joy of my recovery, they talked for a long time about the danger of death in which I had supposedly been."

Since this time, Adler remembers, "that I always imagined my future as a doctor. That is, I set a goal from which I could expect that it could end my childish distress, my fear of death. It is clear that I expected more from this career choice than it could deliver: to overcome death, the fear of death, I should not have expected from human achievements…" (Adler 1986, p. 120).

3.2 Family Situation

In Adler's family, there is a cosmopolitan, optimistic climate. Although the Adlers are Jews, they avoid—as is common among many Viennese Jews—ghettoizing themselves from the environment and moving only in Jewish circles.

This is also related to the fact that faith and religion are given little importance in the Adlers. This is also shown by the fact that Alfred Adler converted to Protestantism much later (in 1904), although he is actually an atheist.

In general, Alfred, despite his initial physical problems, is an unconcerned, open, sociable, and warm-hearted person. He quickly makes friends and develops self-confidence and optimism early on.

The relationship with his mother is described as not quite simple. He had some irrational resentment towards her, which is shown in a striving "away from the mother", in a drive for activity: "I did not like to stay at home because I was not on the best terms with my mother," he writes.

In contrast, the relationship with his father, who is experienced as brave and diligent, is consistently positive.

Dr. Kurt Adler (born 1905), the son of Alfred Adler, who lived in New York until his death, just like his sister Alexandra, and worked as a doctor and individual psychologist (for many years he was also president of the International Association for Individual Psychology), told me in an interview I conducted with him in the 1980s:

> **Interview**
>
> "Firstly, I can remember that my father often told that as a four-year-old or five-year-old he always went for walks with his father in the morning. Very early, at 5 o'clock or 6 o'clock in the morning. And that his father told him: 'Alfred, don't believe anything!' That doesn't mean that he shouldn't have any faith, but that he should always check everything to see if it's true, and he shouldn't just believe everything."

3.3 School, Studies, and Start of Career

Alfred may be his father's favorite son, but he is only an average student. He particularly struggles with mathematics and drawing. As a result, he has to repeat a year in high school. He barely manages to pass his final exams and enrolls in medical school.

When he graduates in medicine at the age of 25 in 1895, his childhood dream of becoming a doctor comes true. He works in a hospital for 2 years and then opens a private practice—first as an ophthalmologist, later as an internist and neurologist.

His practice is located in the 2nd district in Vienna's Leopoldstadt, where many of his patients live in poor conditions. This reinforces his belief that the Viennese population needs social medical care.

3.4 Starting a Family

At the age of 27, he marries Raissa in 1897, the daughter of a Russian merchant. They later have four children together.

His two children Kurt and Alexandra, who both worked as individual psychologists in New York, described their father in an interview with me as very loving:

> **Interview**
>
> "He was a wonderful father to us children. We always felt that if anything was bad or we had any problem—we could discuss everything with him." (Alexandra)
>
> "My father never forced any of his four children to do anything. He was interested in it, but he did not force me in any direction. ... He was always helpful. He was helpful to all people. The only time he turned away was when someone acted unethically. ... And he always encouraged his patients to act in the sense of a community feeling." (Kurt)

3.5 Freud—Adler

In 1902, Adler is invited by Freud—whose psychoanalytic theses he had defended at the Vienna Medical Association—to the "Psychological Wednesday Society", which only a few psychoanalysts in Vienna attend.

He enjoys the highest recognition among the participants, especially after the publication of his book *Study on the Inferiority of Organs* (1907). Wittels, who also participates in the Wednesday Society, describes him as a stocky and burly man who threw his systematic thoughts into the intricately entwined net of Freudian mechanisms: "I still see him at the round table, the eternal Virginia in his mouth, using the comfortable dialect of the Viennese citizen, as he kept coming back to his idea of the 'inferiority of organs'." (Rattner 1972, p. 22).

Adler despises any pose of authority—especially later on. In this respect, he is almost an "anti-Freud".

3.6 Setting Variables

This is also evident in the setting of the therapist-patient relationship: While in psychoanalysis the patient lies on the couch and the therapist sits behind him in a chair (a clearly hierarchical setting), in individual psychology the patient and therapist sit opposite each other at eye level.

While Freud—according to his own statements—finds it hard to be looked at by patients all day, Adler is an equal, direct counterpart that shows itself. While Freud likes to radiate a magical-mystical aura of omniscience,

Adler is seen as a typical Viennese who presents himself as he is, without any facade.

3.7 Separation

This lively and warm-hearted man soon separates from Freud. He has always felt more drawn to the workers and socialists than to the bourgeois-stiff etiquette of the Freudians. However, the official reason for the separation from Freud were theoretical differences that Freud no longer wanted to accept.

The final break occurred in 1911 when Adler gave two lectures in Freud's discussion circle in which he questioned almost everything that constitutes the pillars of Freudian psychoanalysis:

For him, childhood sexuality is not the decisive cause of neuroses, the Oedipus complex is questioned. Not pleasure, but security, recognition, and power are declared by Adler as the main goals of mental activity.

He formulates this in his text "On the Critique of Freud's Sexual Theory of Mental Life".

One can say: Alfred Adler distances himself from Sigmund Freud after 9 years of collaboration in the psychoanalytic Wednesday Society because he rejects Freud's "biological" drive theory and emphasizes a social psychological perspective in depth psychology.

3.8 Individual Psychology

In 1911, Adler began to develop his method, which he called "Individual Psychology". From this point on, individual psychology had its own theoretical structure and for Adler, it was a distinct psychotherapeutic direction. However, pedagogy was just as important to him—in addition to psychotherapy. He founded his own "Association for Free Psychoanalytic Research", which he renamed "Association for Individual Psychology" in 1913.

After separating from Freud, Adler wrote his book *On the Nervous Character* in 1912,—a first summary of the individual psychological perspectives.

He wrote: "The goal of individual psychology is to change the life plan, the life goals of a person and to strengthen the sense of community."

Dr. Kurt Adler on the differences between individual psychology and psychoanalysis:

> **Interview**
>
> "Individual psychology is first and foremost an ego psychology, not an instinct psychology, but an ego psychology. This means that the ego uses all inheritances, drives, etc. to construct its personality.
>
> This of course sounds very contrary to Freud's view, where instinct, sexuality, is the main thing and determines everything …
>
> Individual psychology is an optimistic psychotherapy method, while Freud's psychology is a pessimistic one. In addition, individual psychology is a very social psychology. It says that one cannot understand a person if one does not see him in relation to his social environment, and where he comes from …"

The life pattern that someone lives more or less unconsciously can be changed by individual psychologists through awareness and deliberate influence.

Because the focus of individual psychology is an active life aimed at a goal. According to this, man is not a victim of his unconscious drive fate, but he can—based on his origin, his abilities and his environment—take his life into his own hands, set goals and achieve them—as long as they are realistic.

3.9 Compensation Ability

According to individual psychology, man is not controlled by his drives, but is a free being who has to solve the cultural tasks that life presents to him. Every person is a unique individual who is responsible for his own life. The goal of individual psychology is for him to understand himself psychologically in his entirety: Who am I? What are my strengths, what are my weaknesses? Where do I want to go? What do I want to do with my lifetime?

Injured feelings from childhood lead to a disturbed self-esteem and form the origin of mental disorders and are often associated with a feeling of inferiority and an insufficiently developed sense of belonging and community. A healthy person learns to compensate for this over the course of his life. Because all too often the normal attempts at compensation fail, this leads to "overcompensation", i.e. excessive compensation efforts, which can then lead to mental illnesses with a variety of symptoms. The attempts at compensation, which manifest themselves, for example, in striving for superiority or in avoidance strategies, are unconscious to the person and are revealed in a kind of secret life plan—which can also have something to do with the position of the child in question in the sibling order (see Sect. 3.1).

3.10 Unconscious Life Plan

In individual psychological psychotherapy, this unconscious life plan should therefore be uncovered. The hidden goals and the injured feelings of childhood are made conscious and worked through in individual psychology by intensive revival. This should minimize the feeling of inferiority and enable a healthy self-assessment of one's own strengths and weaknesses.

Methodologically, access to the unconscious is sought—similar to psychoanalysis—through the analysis of the current life situation, but also in repressed childhood memories, dreams and in the transference relationship.

The goal of individual psychology is therefore primarily to recognize and change the life plan and the life goals of a person and to strengthen the sense of community.

3.11 Community Feeling and Life Goal

A central concept of Adler's individual psychology is "community feeling".

Kurt Adler says:

> **Interview**
>
> "Community feeling means overcoming the feeling that one has to be better and stronger than everyone else. This can be seen in the profession, in sexuality, in relationships and in career choice. From this, one can see whether the personality has the community feeling, to work for others and not just for oneself …
>
> Then it is also very important, especially in neurosis theory, that individual psychology always looks at where the person wants to go, what is his intention, where does he want to go? While most other psychological methods always just ask: 'where does the disease come from?', individual psychology asks: 'what does he intend with his disease?'
>
> The goal orientation of every human movement is important—in health and in disease. Both are always goal-oriented. Man cannot move without having some goal in mind."

3.12 Activities

After separating from Freud, Adler becomes active on many levels: in 1913 he publishes his work *Healing and Educating* and in 1914 the *International Journal for Individual Psychology* is published for the first time. And he increasingly distances himself from Freud:

"Don't worry too much about Freud's chicken coop and his clucking … Since the first significant writings of its builder, the best they (the psychoanalysts) could do was to cluck and re-cluck what we have discussed." (Hoffmann 1997, p. 83).

3.13 Educational Counseling Centers and Children's Clinics

From 1914-1916, Adler serves as a military doctor in Krakow, Brno, and Vienna. After the war, he publishes *The Other Side—A Mass Psychological Study on the Guilt of the People*.

When he returns from the war to Vienna, he establishes a network of about 30 psychotherapeutic educational counseling centers and becomes the chief physician of the first clinic for child psychology in Vienna.

Dr. Alexandra Adler (born 1901), herself a psychiatrist and individual psychologist (from 1954 she was president of the International Association for Individual Psychology), recalls the early days of the educational counseling centers and clinics when she was still studying and in medical training:

> **Interview**
>
> "I often went there when my father was running the clinic. I can remember typical cases where the parents came and said to my father, 'What a terrible boy, he no longer speaks to us, he destroys everything and does not obey us.' My father just listened …
>
> And when the boy came in and just looked at the floor and didn't speak, my father quietly said to him, 'How old do you think I am?' The boy suddenly looked up and started talking to him because he didn't expect that. He expected the doctor to tell him that he is very bad. Instead, my father was very nice to him. And the boy opened up and talked to him. He then told my father that he knows he does things he shouldn't do, and in the future, the boy was usually very cooperative."

3.14 Adler's Image of Humanity

In the interview, Alexandra Adler describes the image of humanity of individual psychologists:

> **Interview**
>
> "Human beings are not naturally evil. No matter what transgressions a person may have committed, misled by his erroneous opinion of life, it need not oppress him. He can change. The past is dead. He is free to be happy and to please others."

Thus, Adler, in his very human approach—not only with children—provides significant impulses for the development of psychotherapy and pedagogy. In so-called outpatient clinics, marriage, family, and sexual counseling are carried out for the first time, and approaches to group therapy are tested. Thus, not only the first Viennese educational counseling centers are created at Adler's suggestion, but their concept is adopted and further developed in the USA, England, and Germany.

3.15 Educational Ideas in "Red Vienna"

These educational counseling centers and children's clinics are run according to the pedagogical ideas and concepts of individual psychology, but these concepts have many similarities with social democratic and socialist educational ideals. And this leads to a number of close cooperations in "Red Vienna" with left-wing organizations for Adler.

It is therefore only understandable that both Social Democrats and liberal Socialists frequent Adler's house. Since Alfred Adler's wife Raissa is Russian and a close friend of Trotsky's wife, Leo Trotsky and other Socialists occasionally appear in Adler's house. Alexandra Adler says in the interview:

> **Interview**
>
> "My parents were not connected with Communists, at least not my father. And the Social Democratic government in Vienna did promote the children's education clinics. There was Glöckl, he was a Social Democrat, there was Sperber and the socialist emphasized ones. And my father also said: 'We are all for the sense of community. And as long as the Socialists emphasize that, they can go with us. But we are not a political direction.' ... Trotsky and Joffe, those are people who left Russia and sat around in the Viennese coffee houses and also visited us at home. ... I remember little of Trotsky—more of his wife and the two children."

3.16 Publications and Lecture Tours

In addition to establishing educational counseling centers and a lectureship at the Vienna Pedagogium, Adler published a series of books from 1921 onwards, such as *Practice and Theory of Individual Psychology* (a collection of lectures), *Understanding Human Nature*—one of his most popular books—and as a late work *The Meaning of Life*, in which he highlights the conflict between subjective meaning and objective sense.

From the 1920s onwards, Alfred Adler often spent half the year restlessly traveling on lecture tours, congresses, and seminars at various universities. His goal is to make individual psychology known in as many countries as possible—including Sweden, Great Britain, the Netherlands, and especially the USA. There, he has held a visiting professorship at Columbia University in New York since 1926. By the early 1930s, Adler was considered one of the most famous psychologists in the Western world. His son, Kurt Adler, recalls:

> **Interview**
>
> "My father always believed that he had to spread individual psychology. And that's why he traveled so much to give lectures everywhere. And psychological groups were then also formed in these countries, in Holland, in England and later also in America. … In America, he also held weekly meetings with his closer individual psychologists."

3.17 Relocation to the USA

Even in the years before he fully moved to the USA, Adler usually spent half a year in Europe and the other half in the USA.

In 1934, he moved his residence entirely to New York, along with several family members, where he had been lecturing at Columbia University in New York for many years. In 1935, he founded the American edition of the *International Journal of Individual Psychology*.

But after the Nazis took power in Germany, he no longer felt drawn back to the European mainland—at best, he still traveled to Great Britain. And that was his last trip in 1937. Alexandra Adler says in an interview:

> **Interview**
>
> "Since Vienna, he was very depressed because my older sister, when Hitler came, had fled with all German colleagues to Russia. Under Stalin, all these Germans were arrested, my sister too—and we never heard from her again. She was banished without any trial. We tried everything. My father even tried to do something through Roosevelt, but she was not an American citizen and no one could help her.
>
> When my father went to Great Britain at that time, I came to him to say goodbye, and I told him: 'If you go to Great Britain now, maybe my sister will soon be with you.' I didn't believe it myself, but I wanted to cheer him up because he was so depressed. The last words I heard from him were: 'I just wish it was already so far …'"

3.18 Last Days

Alfred Adler, then 67 years old, is in Scotland—always committed to his individual psychology—to hold a lecture series at the University of Aberdeen. The night before, he goes to the cinema with the Bottome couple (Phyllis B. later becomes his biographer) to watch the film "The Great Barrier". Afterwards, he writes a series of letters and postcards.

As usual for him as an early riser, he goes for a morning walk in the park on Union Street before his lecture at the university. A girl is said to have seen him on this walk and thought: "What a strong old man: He takes steps like an athlete."

Suddenly he stumbles, collapses and falls. Since he can no longer get up on his own, a student comes to help. Resuscitation attempts, heart massages are tried. Adler still calls for his son Kurt. Then acute heart failure sets in and Alfred Adler dies of a heart attack. It is May 28, 1937, around 9:15 a.m.

Alfred Adler dies without warning, seemingly out of the blue. The restlessness, which sometimes became hectic, is also reflected in his way of dying.

And indeed, in Adler's work, death and dying are given little space. While "finality" (goal orientation) and "lifestyle" are central terms in individual psychology, dealing with death is not one of the central themes in this optimistic, life-affirming therapy method. And this is not least reflected in the way Alfred Adler dies.

Alexandra Adler says in an interview:

> **Interview**
>
> "Our friends saw him when he was dead, and when they put him on the stretcher, he made a movement as if he would help them, as he always did. And that was the last thing we heard."

3.19 Cremation and Honorary Grave in Vienna

Death unfortunately has the ability to remind itself at the most inconvenient moments: Alfred Adler dies unexpectedly at the age of 67 from a heart attack in the Scottish city of Aberdeen. His body is cremated in Edinburgh. Although his family travels to the funeral, the urn remains in the Warriston crematorium in Edinburgh.

Only in 2009 is it sought by the Association for Individual Psychology, brought to Vienna with the help of an honorary consul in April 2011, and on July 12, 2011–74 years after his death—it is buried in an honorary grave at the Vienna Central Cemetery.

3.20 The Social Genius

Alfred Adler, whom the writer Manés Sperber calls "the social genius", is the founder of a psychotherapy direction, whose insights appear again and again in many other psychotherapy schools, but are hardly associated with individual psychology or with Alfred Adler.

It is like a late revenge of Freud's that most of Adler's insights are attributed to him, Sigmund Freud.

3.21 Conclusion

Alfred Adler maintains a rather casual, relaxed approach to himself, other people, and the world in his life. The life-loving, socially committed, warm-hearted helper type, the representative of an "optimistic psychology", becomes hectic when it comes to the development and dissemination of his method.

In individual psychology, which rather puts the future goal orientation in the foreground than dealing with the past, the confrontation with death and the preparation for dying do not play a central role. Adler therefore tirelessly travels through America and Europe to spread his individual psychology, and succumbs—completely unexpectedly and without a long death struggle—to a heart attack in a park in Aberdeen, Scotland.

Bibliography

Adler, Alfred: Menschenkenntnis, Frankfurt 1986 (Fischer)
Hoffmann, Edward: Alfred Adler, München 1997 (Reinhardt)
Rattner, Josef: Alfred Adler, Reinbek 1972 (rororo-Monographien)

Further Reading

Adler, Alfred: Praxis und Theorie der Individualpsychologie, Darmstadt (1969)
Adler, Alfred: Über den nervösen Charakter, Darmstadt (1969)
Adler, Alfred: Der Sinn des Lebens, München 1987
Jacoby, Henry: Alfred Adler – Individualpsychologie und dialektische Charakterkunde Frankfurt 1983 (Fischer-TB)
Kluy, Alexander: Alfred Adler, München 2019 (DVA)
Sperber, Manes: Alfred Adler oder: Das Elend der Psychologie, Berlin 1983 (Ullstein)
Interview mit Dr. Alexandra und Dr. Kurt Adler, den beiden Kindern von Alfred Adler (1985)

4

Interlude II: On Dying

Contents

4.1 Death as the Great Equalizer 36
4.2 A Fairy Tale 36
Further Reading 37

> This is about the general topic of dying—situated between scientific knowledge, idealization, and banality, it affects us all. Death spares no one. We don't have to learn to die, we all manage it—somehow.

Death smiles at us all. The only thing you can do is smile back. (Marcus Aurelius)

To consider, **that** we die, makes one wise, says a biblical Psalm. **How** we die, scares some people. Writing about the death of great psychotherapists may seem delicate to many—and it is.

Scientific language is inappropriate in the face of death. A too emotional language may not maintain the necessary distance. Thus, the whole thing—like so much in life—is a tightrope walk. On the one hand, there is the danger of falling into uncritical glorification, embellishment, exaltation, and idealization of these outstanding individuals—as is not uncommon among adepts and especially biographers of the respective psychotherapists.

On the other hand, the abyss of the banal beckons.

4.1 Death as the Great Equalizer

With great people, many believe, everything is grand. Everything is so grand that the ordinary would be too small—including their way of dying. It's good that the deceased (with great probability) do not know what is said about them after their death, what has happened to them.

In fact, death is the great equalizer. And it connects us all with these individuals. Because it takes them all—the poor and the rich, the wise and the foolish, the men and the women, the young and the old, the powerful and the powerless. Perhaps there is something comforting in this, our commonality: No one comes out of life alive. And yet, dying is something highly individual—because everyone dies their own death in their very personal way.

We don't have to learn to die, we can all die—each in his own way, very individually: whether dramatically or quietly, elegantly or clumsily, whether painfully or lightly, full of pain or flowing into redemption.

Basically, we don't need a "last aid course": We all manage it, at most we can perhaps make dying easier for ourselves with external help. Because dealing with it is not easy—neither with one's own death nor with the death of others. But we cannot escape it. Because death is omnipresent around us, but we have no influence on our fate and therefore on him. A wonderful Arabic fairy tale tells of this, which I would like to offer you for comfort.

4.2 A Fairy Tale

"Sultan, I beg you, lend me your fastest horse. I must ride to Damascus immediately." The Sultan's gardener had stormed up the steps of the palace in Baghdad. "What has happened, what makes you so excited?"

"My Sultan," the gardener replied agitatedly, "just now I met death in the garden. He raised his arms and threatened me. That's why I absolutely have to get away from here. Because far away from here, in Damascus, I will be safe."

Since the Sultan valued his gardener, he did not hesitate and gave the gardener his best horse. The gardener swung himself onto the horse and rode as fast as he could.

The Sultan went into the garden, where he indeed found the Grim Reaper. He asked Death: "Why are you threatening my faithful gardener?"

Death shook his head. "No, I did not threaten your gardener. I was just surprised myself." The Sultan retorted: "Don't make excuses, you scared him to death."

"Really, no," replied the Grim Reaper, "I just clapped my hands over my head because I was surprised to see the gardener here in Baghdad. Because my order was to take him far away from here, in Damascus, tonight."

Further Reading

Mauder, Albert: Die Kunst des Sterbens, Regensburg 1976 (Pustet)
Hampe, Johann-Christoph: Sterben ist doch ganz anders, Stuttgart 1975 (Kreuz)
Langbein, Kurt, Skalnik, Christian: Leben verlängern – um welchen Preis? München 1996 (Europa)
Nuland, Sherwin B.: Wie wir sterben, München 1996 (Knaur)
Schüle, Christian: Wie wir sterben lernen, München 2013 (Pattloch)
Tausch, Anna-Marie + Reinhard: Sanftes Sterben, Reinbek 1985 (Rowohlt)

5

Wilhelm Reich (1897–1957): Destruction of a Heretic

Contents

5.1	Emotional Illiterates	41
5.2	"Emotional Plague"	41
5.3	Inner World Pollution	42
5.4	Libido Theory	42
5.5	Childhood and Youth	43
5.6	Psychoanalysis	44
5.7	The Function of the Orgasm	45
5.8	Psychoanalysis and Marxism	45
5.9	Character Analysis	46
5.10	Emigration	46
5.11	Orgone I	47
5.12	From Libido to Bioenergy	47
5.13	Armorings	48
5.14	Practice	48
5.15	Physiology and Psychology	48
5.16	Orgone Therapy	49
5.17	Scandinavia—USA	50
5.18	Savior	50
5.19	Orgon II	50
5.20	Einstein	51
5.21	Charlatanism and Persecution	51
5.22	Destruction of the Life's Work	52
5.23	Prison and Death	52
5.24	Conclusion	53
Bibliography		53

© The Author(s), under exclusive license to Springer-Verlag GmbH, DE, part of Springer Nature 2024
W. Gross, *As One Lives, So One Dies*, https://doi.org/10.1007/978-3-662-70061-7_5

> **Trailer**
>
> This chapter is about Wilhelm Reich, the revolutionary, the alternative, the heretic, and the activist. He is another dissident of psychoanalysis. He has set himself the goal of liberating the soul through work on the body. Over the course of his professional development, he moves further and further away from psychoanalysis, first establishing character analysis and later orgone therapy. He has to flee into exile in other countries several times before settling in the USA. But even there he is not safe, as his work is not accepted, but fought against.
>
> He dies—whether he has gone mad or not—in prison a kind of "self-death", as he has to watch his entire life's work being destroyed by the state. In a sense, he suffers the fate of many politically persecuted people and simply gives up at some point.

One starts life as an arsonist—and ends it as a firefighter. (Pittigrilli)

> Wilhelm Reich is considered one of the most fascinating, but also one of the most controversial psychotherapists of the therapy founder generation. He was a doctor, psychoanalyst, and social revolutionary, a cancer cell biologist and peace philosopher, a communist and bestselling author, founder of the Sex-Pol movement and rainmaker. He was seen as a genius and a madman, as a fantasist and a materialist. To this day, he is revered and admired, rejected and demonized—or ignored.

Wilhelm Reich, the founder of character analysis, vegetotherapy, and orgone therapy, is primarily known in current psychotherapy for the impulses he has given for the various body psychotherapy methods developed by his later students:

- Bioenergetics (Alexander Lowen),
- Biodynamics (Gerda Boyesen),
- Radix Emotional Education (Charles R. Kelley),
- Core Energetics (John Pierrakos),
- Biosynthesis (David Boadella),
- Life Energy Process (Stèphano Sabetti).

Reich is thus something like the progenitor of depth psychology-based body psychotherapy methods.

His original goal is to further develop psychoanalysis from the pure "talking cure" to the psychosomatic integration of the body into psychotherapy. And this has the following background:

Language is seen in traditional depth psychological psychotherapy approaches not only as a means of mere communication, but also as a possibility to verbalize sensations and self-reflection. "Where Id was, Ego shall be," Sigmund Freud formulated. And for this, language is an important—the central—instrument. This is how Wilhelm Reich also started.

However, Wilhelm Reich saw very early on that there is a not to be overlooked danger in the use of language as an instrument: that it is not only a means of communication, but also per se a defense formation of emotions and sensory impressions.

More and more people, it seems, live more in a "word world" than in sensual reality. Thus, every verbal expression already acknowledges the reified, emotion-stripped symbolic language. This danger naturally comes to light particularly in therapeutic schools where words represent the main psychotherapeutic instrument.

5.1 Emotional Illiterates

"Man lives through the head," Bert Brecht had already complained in a song in the 1920s—exactly at the time when psychoanalysis was gaining importance. And this had a societal background then as it does today, because the fear of physical contact in our Central European regions was and is proverbial. In everyday life, adults do not touch each other—especially now again in (post-)Corona times—unless during sexual experiences, aggressive confrontations, or at the doctor's. It is only logical that many experience themselves as physical and emotional illiterates.

5.2 "Emotional Plague"

Wilhelm Reich called these deserts within us the "emotional plague": From the originally life-loving and spontaneous human being, a constricted, compulsively reacting personality develops over the course of life, suppressing all spontaneous feelings, living passionless and affectless like an automaton.

From the outside, this is rarely noticeable. He is well adapted socially, the facade is intact: shapely, shockproof, breakproof, and washable. He reacts as expected of him: mechanically, superficially, nicely. In his job, he meets the expectations of his employer, is a "good" worker, employee, or staff member.

He treats his body just as mechanistically: It has to function, just like the car, the refrigerator, the washing machine, the mobile phone, the iPad.

Increasingly, the "appendage" body becomes less of an opportunity to experience intense pleasure and meaning. As if amputated from his physicality, he continues to live, and the body (which he once could feel with pleasure and pain) becomes more and more of a phantom to him. Any kind of feeling and experiencing (physical and emotional) seems foreign to him. He feels empty and alienated.

5.3 Inner World Pollution

Just as there is environmental pollution, there is inner world pollution. According to Reich, it is a kind of "flirtation with death" that makes one susceptible to mental and physical diseases.

The fight against the "dull nature", against the "beast in man", is not only a creeping destruction of physicality, it is simultaneously the destruction of emotional life and the inner nature of man—so Reich's view.

With the loss of his sensuality, he has also lost his sense. This is also related to the suppression of any natural sexuality, which—if you practice it long enough – then only dares to express itself in absurd fantasies or sexual perversions.

And if not at some point an "inexplicable" physical or mental illness appears and punches a hole in the facade, nobody would notice:

"Actually, I am quite different. But I rarely get the chance to be so", the Austro-Hungarian writer Ödön von Horvath described the situation. This is the social background that Reich tried to change at various levels throughout his life.

5.4 Libido Theory

Psychoanalysis had once started quite differently. Freud (together with Breuer) began to work psychotherapeutically with hypnosis in 1887. At that time, the goal was to evoke traumatic memories, which were accompanied by strong cathartic discharges and involved the entire body, where in the "abreaction" both physical and psychological energies were released. The patients cried, screamed, raged in the therapy session—and usually felt liberated afterwards. However, the change only lasted for a short time, and the patients showed the old symptoms again. Therefore, he developed the psychoanalytic methods still in use today (free association, basic rule, insight into the disease through interpretation and analysis).

His "**libido theory**" was originally an energy concept. Freud wrote about this in 1914:

"It may be, if we penetrate far and deep, that we discover that the sexual energy, the libido, is only the diverse product of an energy working generally in the brain."

Until then, Freud was still heavily involved with energetic processes in psychoanalysis. The energy that showed itself in the emotions and symptoms of his patients, Freud considered as "something that is capable of increasing, decreasing, shifting, discharging and extending itself along the memory paths of a thought, like an electrical charge over the surface of a body".

And the original goal of Freud's therapeutic work was to free the "trapped affect" that hides behind the symptoms. He retains this goal, but psychoanalysis becomes more and more a conversation. The body no longer serves as a means of expression, psychoanalysis becomes more and more a "language game" (Lorenzer). And that is exactly what Reich tries to change in the course of his development. He wants to put the head back on its feet, so to speak, by granting the body (and thus the emotions) its space. His credo is well formulated in a text by Vladimir Iljine:

If I have lost my body, I have lost myself. If I find my body, I find myself. If I move, I live and move the world. Without this body I am not—and as my body I am. Only in movement do I experience myself as my body -my body experiences itself, I experience myself. My body is the coincidence of being and knowledge, of subject and object. It is the starting point and the end of my existence.

5.5 Childhood and Youth

Wilhelm Reich was born on March 24, 1897 in Galicia. His parents are assimilated Jews, who deny little Wilhelm both contact with Jewish-speaking children and with the peasant children from the surrounding area.

Soon after Wilhelm's birth, the family moves to Bukovina, a border area between Central, Southern and Eastern Europe, which at that time still belonged to the Habsburg monarchy of Austria-Hungary.

The father, Leon Reich, acquires a large farm, where he mainly breeds cattle. When Wilhelm is 3 years old, his brother Robert is born.

Until he goes to the German-speaking grammar school in Czernowitz, he is essentially left to himself and is only taught by private tutors.

A dramatic cut in Wilhelm's life happens when his mother commits suicide in 1910. He is 13 years old at this time. The (suspected) reason:

Allegedly, Wilhelm betrayed his extremely jealous father about his mother's affair with a private tutor. However, not much is known about this.

Four years later, in 1914, the father dies of tuberculosis and Wilhelm has to manage the entire estate alone at the age of 17.

After he completes his Matura (high school diploma) in 1915, he is drafted for military service in the Austrian army.

After the end of World War I, he has lost his estate in the chaos of war. He goes quite impoverished to his brother in Vienna, who—because he was too young for military service during the war—has been living there for a longer time and provides for the livelihood of the two in the first semesters. Wilhelm begins to study law, but switches to medicine in the winter semester of 1918/1919.

5.6 Psychoanalysis

Relatively early on, he developed an interest in psychoanalysis, organizing a "Student Seminar for Sexology" as early as 1919, meeting Sigmund Freud for the first time that year, and treating his first patient using the psychoanalytic method.

He developed such an interest and energy for psychoanalysis that he was admitted to the Vienna Psychoanalytic Society on October 13, 1920.

He was just 23 years old and was considered a brilliant thinker, eloquent participant in discussions, and author of theoretical articles on psychoanalytic topics, even among much older psychoanalysts.

His first psychoanalytic work was titled *Ibsen's Peer Gynt—Libido Conflicts and Delusions*.

He began a training analysis with Paul Federn, which he did not complete.

In 1921, he married his fellow student, Annie Pink, and completed his medical studies a year later as Dr. med.

His daughter Eva was born in 1924, who would later manage his estate.

Although Freud rejected Reich's wish to complete his training analysis with him, he soon received patients directly from Freud and took over—at just 27 years old—the direction of the "Seminar for Psychoanalytic Therapy".

His brother Robert died of tuberculosis in 1926, and Wilhelm also had to undergo treatment for a lung condition in Davos, Switzerland. This stay in the sanatorium probably also helped him to intensify the inclusion of the body in the psychoanalytic process.

5.7 The Function of the Orgasm

In 1927, he published his controversially discussed book *The Function of the Orgasm*. His theory—still entirely in the jargon of psychoanalysis—states that the restricted orgasmic surrender forms the energetic basis of neurosis. It is critically questioned by many psychoanalysts. Nevertheless, the book makes him known worldwide among colleagues—although the reaction of the psychoanalytic colleagues continues to be divided and ranges from recognition and admiration to strong rejection. Even Freud reacts with irritation. When he presented the manuscript to him on the occasion of Freud's 70th birthday with the dedication "To my teacher, Prof. Sigmund Freud, with deep reverence", Freud only said, irritated: "So thick?"

Already in this book, Reich lays the foundation for the questions that he never loses sight of throughout his life:

What are the fundamental biological drives? What is the energy of life and the living? What are their functions and laws of function?

When his second daughter Lore is born in 1928, Reich becomes more involved in the socialist party for communist ideas and founds the "Socialist Society for Social Counseling". This also reflects Reich's insight that mental illnesses are not only an individual problem but also a societal one.

Therefore, the counseling centers should primarily work prophylactically through education. Here also grows his love for the working class, which he considers healthier than the bourgeoisie.

5.8 Psychoanalysis and Marxism

Over time, he increasingly moved away from the orthodox psychoanalytic method and tried to connect Marxism and psychoanalysis.

In 1929, Reich went on a lecture and study trip in the USSR. He returned disappointed that the sexual reform in the land of the revolution was inadequately implemented—or even withdrawn.

Although he remained a member of the Communist Party, he was very dissatisfied with this in Vienna and moved to Berlin, where the Communists were much stronger. Even there in the psychoanalytic society, he felt increasingly uncomfortable—although he found like-minded conversation partners in Otto Fenichel, Erich Fromm, and Karen Horney.

He developed a sexual political platform that formed the basis for the later Sex-Pol movement, which was successful in the 1930s and was later picked up again by the 68 student movement.

Overall, however, his attempted bridge between psychoanalysis and Marxism failed, and he was more or less expelled from both ideological directions.

Wilhelm Reich had to flee Germany in 1933 because the Nazis had taken power in Berlin and he was Jewish. In addition, his marriage to Annie, which had been faltering for years, failed.

5.9 Character Analysis

When he published the first version of the *Character Analysis* in Denmark in 1933, this book brought him great recognition among followers of psychoanalysis, and he managed to gather students and followers around him once again in Copenhagen. However, he was also expelled from the Communist Party in Denmark—probably because his ideas about sexual liberation did not fit into the concept of the local CP. And his standing in the psychoanalytic community also became increasingly difficult.

5.10 Emigration

Despite this, he remains very active professionally and the ballet dancer Elsa Lindenberg, whom he had already met in Berlin, becomes his life partner—until his emigration to the USA in 1939.

When his residence permit is not extended in Denmark, he first goes to Sweden, but there too they do not want the "troublemaker". He initially moves on to the Norwegian capital Oslo, where he acts less politically and devotes himself more and more to the connection between psyche and body in psychotherapy.

For him, from then on there is a close connection between "character armor" and "muscle armor". And when the muscle armor is broken up,—according to Reich's opinion—"libido" is released.

In Oslo, starting in 1935, he begins to move further away from psychoanalysis as a therapy method, and becomes more and more involved with general energetic processes in living organisms. In his "splendid isolation" he creates his own "world explanation systems". In bion research, which is difficult to understand for the uninitiated, he then discovers the life energy, which he calls "orgone".

5.11 Orgone I

Reich views a person from a holistic energetic and biological perspective. He sees humans in all their aspirations as a biological being that basically reacts like **an** organism, like **a** cell. And he finds that for every mental illness there is a correlate in the patient's body, i.e. an "identity of psychic ego structure and physical constitution". So it is only logical that he overcomes the touch taboo of psychoanalysis and approaches both the "muscle armor" of the patient physically and the "character armor" psychotherapeutically. He initially calls this "character analysis", then "vegetotherapy" and later "orgone therapy".

5.12 From Libido to Bioenergy

Later, Reich expands the libido concept to a bioenergy concept, the energy of which he calls "orgone" (derived from "organism" and "orgasm").

Therapy according to Reich is therefore work on the body and with the feelings. It is rooted in the two main discoveries of Wilhelm Reich:

The first is the muscle armor (the chronic tension patterns in the body that are responsible for blocked feelings).

The second is the life energy that can be felt in the body, which serves as a bridging concept between the armor and the blocked feelings.

Another main thought of Reich refers to the role of sexuality for the regulation of the energy balance in the body.

Reich believes that a full orgasmic satisfaction breaks down all excess energy in the organism and that no energy remains in the body to support neurotic behavior patterns. This is therefore the function of the orgasm: the reduction of physical and psychological tensions.

If the energy is held in chronic muscle tensions, this reduction is not possible. Therefore, these must be eliminated if the full orgasm is to be achieved. Reich was convinced that if a person develops the ability to break down all his excess energy in orgasm, i.e. if he becomes orgasmically potent, then his emotional health is assured, because then no energy is available for neurotic patterns. Therefore, orgasmic potency becomes Reich's therapeutic goal.

5.13 Armorings

Character analysis could still be accommodated in the Freudian system—all later methods could not. Completely new and revolutionary are Reich's discoveries in the field of the autonomic nervous system and the muscular armorings arranged in a ring around the body axis. He had thus—uninfluenced by Far Eastern methods—almost found an equivalent to the "chakras" that play an important role in yoga.

Orgone therapists and bioenergetics distinguish—like Reich himself—various "muscle segments" in the body, in which "armorings" preferably settle:

- In the upper half of the head, especially the eye zone and the forehead,
- the lower part of the head, especially the mouth and jaw,
- neck and throat (as one of the two main constrictions of the body),
- chest and upper back,
- waist/diaphragm (as the second main constriction of the body),
- abdomen,
- pelvis.

5.14 Practice

The client lies lightly dressed on a couch or mattress, so that the therapist can appropriately observe and treat his reactions and his condition. There are in
the orgone therapy three important approaches to the patient:

1. The breathing,
2. the direct manipulation of cramped muscles,
3. the psychotherapeutic work according to the character-analytical method.

5.15 Physiology and Psychology

Reich thus combines physiology with psychology (which was originally also the goal of psychoanalysis), by viewing humans holistically and solving the mind-body problem in this way. He can be seen—not only on this level—as a kind of "pioneer". After Freud abandoned the energy-economic approach,

Reich not only took over his libido theory, but expanded it to the orgone theory. Reich writes:

"Freud's authors simply referred to the term libido as the unconscious desire for sexual acts."

For Freud, libido is a word of consciousness psychology. Reich believes that Freud did not really know what libido was or should be. Freud meant: We can't really grasp the drive. What we experience are only derivatives of the drive, sexual ideas and affects. The drive itself rests deep in the biological basis of the organism and manifests itself as an affective urge for satisfaction. We feel the urge for relaxation, but not the drive itself …

Reich interprets Freud as follows: "It is perfectly logical that the drive itself cannot be conscious, for it is what governs and controls us. We are its object. … Just as electricity becomes measurable through its energy manifestations, so drives are only recognizable through affect manifestations. Freud's libido means the conscious sexual desire that one feels. Freud's libido is and can be nothing other than the energy of the sexual drive."

5.16 Orgone Therapy

The orgone therapy is closely linked to the biological energy that Reich calls "orgone". Simply put: If enough "orgone energy" freely and strongly pulses through the body, then the person is considered healthy and feels good. If this energy is blocked, the person in question first feels uncomfortable and later develops mental and/or physical diseases. The goal of orgone therapy is therefore to eliminate these energy blockages in the body, so that the energy can flow freely again and thus the mental state of the patient is better.—His psyche is then also free of blockages, inhibitions and disturbances. Because the "body armor" inhibits the free flow of energy in the organism together with the psychological "character armor". Energy that cannot be discharged accumulates and forms "stasis energy", which (according to Reich) leads to blockages as static energy and manifests itself in symptoms.

The fact that Reich touches his patients in orgone therapy and tries to physically dissolve energy blocks finally separates him from classical psychoanalysis with its taboo on touch. Reich believes that the central task of orgone therapy is the "destruction of armor", in other words the restoration of the mobility of the body plasma. Because in the armored organism, the pulsation function in all organs is more or less restricted. The goal of orgone therapy is to restore the full ability to pulsate. The result of ideally performed orgone therapy is the occurrence of the orgasm reflex. According to Reich, it is, next to breathing, the most important movement phenomenon in the animal kingdom. The organism "gives itself" completely to its organ sensations and involuntary body convulsions at the moment of orgasm. Because the movement of the orgasm reflex is associated with the expression of "surrender".

5.17 Scandinavia—USA

In 1937, still in Scandinavia, he meets the educator Alexander S. Neill, the later founder of "anti-authoritarian education", which he tested in the British Summerhill School. Neill writes:

"I am quite sure that the difference between Reich and all the scientists I have met lay in his extraordinary vitality, his awareness, his humanity."

The bion research and rumors about Reich's earlier sexual therapy methods are blown up in a discriminatory press campaign in Norway against him, so that he feels compelled to emigrate to the USA in 1939.

The fact that he has a contract as an associate professor at the New School for Social Research in New York makes his renewed emigration easier.

Full of optimism, he sets up his own laboratory in New York, hoping that the USA is open to his new findings.

There he also meets Ilse Ollendorf, who initially becomes his assistant. He marries her at the end of 1939 and she remains his companion until 1954. It seems as if Reich, in order to be professionally productive, always needs a partner at his side. Their son Peter is born in 1944.

5.18 Savior

Reich is a tireless "hard worker": In addition to his research, he gives lectures, has students again and successfully treats patients. Thus, he gathers a few admirers around him who see him as the savior who solves all the problems of life for them. However, he refuses to seek official medical certification. This will later be his downfall.

5.19 Orgon II

"Orgon" is for Wilhelm Reich a kind of general life energy that exists in all living things. Since the 1940s, he has been moving away from pure psychotherapy, especially since he has been living in the USA, towards the exploration of general life processes. During this time, he develops strange devices to concentrate the life energy "Orgon". It is these "Orgon accumulations", "Orgon engines", "Orgon shooters" and "Cloud-Busters" that later become his downfall.

As early as 1940, he built the first "Orgon Accumulator", a cabinet-like box in which the life energy "Orgon" is supposed to accumulate in particularly high concentration. Spending time in it daily, in his view, not only cures diseases but also prevents them.

5.20 Einstein

Reich also reports this new discovery to Albert Einstein in a letter. Einstein invites him for talks in 1941, but after initially showing interest, he no longer wants to know anything about Reich's discoveries. Reich is outraged by Einstein's behavior and suspects a communist conspiracy behind it, later calling it the "Einstein Affair".

In 1946, Reich becomes a US citizen and moves his laboratory from New York to a property near Rangley/Maine, which he calls "Orgonon", where he works and conducts all his experiments. He begins building an observatory, which later serves as his workplace. In 1948, the first international orgonomic congress is held at Orgonon.

5.21 Charlatanism and Persecution

Similar to Norway, after some time there is again a concerted press campaign against him, triggered in 1947 by an article by journalist Mildred Brady in the magazine *New Republic*. The Food and Drug Administration (FDA), a US health agency, systematically tries to obstruct and ban work with the "Orgon Accumulators".

In addition, in 1950 Reich's not exactly harmless Oranur experiments to explore the relationship between Orgon and nuclear radiation and his attempts to influence the weather with the help of a "Cloud-Buster". The accusation: charlatanism.

Over the next few years, the campaign against Reich takes on increasingly worse forms. As Reich sees the destruction of his life's work approaching, he feels—rightly or wrongly—persecuted. Over the last years of his life, however, he also develops clear paranoid traits that have little to do with reality. David Boadella, a Reichian and biographer of Reich, writes:

"In the end, however, the paranoid delusion gradually ate into him, silently and treacherously like a mental cancer. The soaring feelings and ideas of his last years were something like a feverish protective reaction against the paralyzing cold of the world rejecting him." (Boadella 1981, p. 305).

5.22 Destruction of the Life's Work

Reich's world gradually collapses like a house of cards: As early as the summer of 1954, Ilse Ollendorf has separated from Reich and he initially starts a relationship with Grete Hoff. Later, Aurora Karrer becomes his life partner, with whom he still makes plans for the future.

Finally, on February 10, 1954, a trial against Reich takes place, which he does not attend. After a 7-year investigation, he is forbidden to continue using and selling Orgon accumulators. Reich does not comply and two years later the court orders the destruction of all Orgon accumulators and all of Reich's specialist literature—including *Mass Psychology of Fascism*, *Character Analysis* and *Speech to the Little Man*. Thus, in 1956, entire truckloads of Reichian scientific literature are consumed by flames in an American waste incineration plant. All equipment is also destroyed under FDA supervision. Son Peter dramatically describes the situation of the destruction of the Orgon accumulators in his book *The Dream Father*, which he had to witness as a 12-year-old. Reich's fears have come true: his life's work is destroyed.

5.23 Prison and Death

He himself is sentenced to 2 years in prison, which he has to start on March 12, 1957. He still hopes for a probation hearing in prison, which is already scheduled for November 10, 1957, and also writes to his wife: "I could not bear prison well and will—very likely—be killed there." (Laska 1981, p. 127).

On November 3, 1957, he is found dead in his bed in the morning.

The death certificate tersely states: "Heart failure: Myocardial insufficiency with sudden cardiac arrest, accompanied by general arteriosclerosis and sclerosis of the coronary vessels". The result of an examination for toxins in the autopsy is negative. He was 61 years old.

Many myths surround Reich's death: from being poisoned or driven to death to a natural death in an unusual situation, the range is wide.

What will remain of him are his suggestions for (body) psychotherapy, the many psychological and (socio-)political publications, the Wilhelm Reich Museum at "Orgonon" and the memories of a dazzling personality.

5.24 Conclusion

Wilhelm Reich, the revolutionary, the politician, the heretic and activist, moves further and further away from psychoanalysis over the course of his professional development.

At first, he only includes the body in psychotherapy, establishes character analysis and later orgone therapy. After that, he deals with general energetic processes. He develops strange devices—orgone accumulators, orgone shooters—experiments with nuclear material and tries to influence the weather.

Over the course of his life, he has to flee into exile in other countries several times before settling in the USA. But even there he is not safe, as his work is not accepted and is fought against.

He dies—whether he has gone mad or not—in prison a kind of "self-death", as he has to watch his entire life's work being destroyed by the state. In a sense, he suffers the fate of many political persecutors and simply gives up at some point.

Bibliography

Boadella, David: Wilhelm Reich, München 1981 (Scherz)
Krieger, Hans: Wilhelm Reich, der Mann, der an unsere tiefsten Ängste rührte, Hamburg, Selbstverlag (ohne Angabe)
Laska, Bernd A.: Wilhelm Reich, Reinbek 1981 (rororo Monographien)
Ollendorff-Reich, Ilse: Wilhelm Reich, München 1975 (Kindler)
Raknes, Ola: Wilhelm Reich und die Orgonomie, Frankfurt 1983 (Nexus)
Reich, Wilhelm: Funktion des Orgasmus, Köln 1987 (Kiepenheuer + Witsch)
Reich, Wilhelm: Charakteranalyse, Frankfurt 1977 (Fischer TB)
Reich, Wilhelm: Die Entdeckung des Orgons Bd. 1 und Bd. 2, Frankfurt 1977 (Fischer TB)

6

Interlude III: The Phases of Dying

Contents

6.1	Denial	56
6.2	Anger	56
6.3	Bargaining	56
6.4	Depression	56
6.5	Acceptance	57
6.6	Individuality	57
Further Reading		58

> This article is about the way we die and how we deal with it. Elisabeth Kübler-Ross divided the psychological confrontation with the process of impending death into five stages of dying. These will be explained in more detail here.

Being dead is (probably) easy. Dying is sometimes hard.

Swiss psychiatrist Elisabeth Kübler-Ross (1926–2004) spent many years studying death and dying. Through her long-term encounters with dying people, she observed five phases of psychological experience in dealing with death:

6.1 Denial

When people receive a lethal diagnosis from a doctor, many are initially shocked. A kind of shock paralysis with numbness and/or physical complaints arises. This shock phase is a protective reaction of the soul. Often associated with it are denial and refusal to accept the reality, because the idea of dying soon seems unbearable to them. Often, those affected isolate themselves in this phase and may not be able to talk about it and cannot think about the consequences—because the shock predominates.

6.2 Anger

Once the initial shock has passed, intense emotions often emerge: anger, rage, resistance, and blame. Sometimes these feelings do not openly surface, but subtly show that one cannot please the person concerned. Often these feelings are also directed against relatives, doctors, and caregivers. They are held responsible for the fate of the dying person and his situation. But there can also be aggression towards one's own "incapable" body—or thoughts of suicide may arise.

6.3 Bargaining

The person concerned tries to negotiate with fate, with themselves, with doctors or (for believers) with God. Sometimes "vows" are then made: "If I make it again, then I will …" He/she hopes for a longer life through good cooperation with the "higher power" and clings to everything that promises healing—the much-cited "last straw". Everything just to escape the danger of death. Sometimes completely unrealistic wishes are expressed in this phase.

6.4 Depression

When it becomes clear to the person concerned that he/she will die, this can be accompanied by intense grief reactions, fears, and depression. Reflections and deep sorrow about the fact that one's own life is really coming to an end are in the foreground. Then what will no longer be possible in the future is mourned: The loss of physical integrity, the loss of personal and professional opportunities, the loss of unfulfilled wishes—the unlived life.

6.5 Acceptance

Accepting what is, is now in the foreground. In the phase of acceptance, the person concerned has accepted their own fate. The facts are accepted by the dying person without ifs and buts. He/she faces fate calmly and settles last matters. This leads to a calm state. Often the need for conversation dries up. The gaze is more inward. The desire to receive visitors decreases. If people can die in this phase, their death is often a gentle falling asleep and "letting go", after they have said goodbye to their important reference persons.

6.6 Individuality

Of course, every dying process is highly individual for the person(s) concerned and not every dying person goes through the phases in this order—and the phases not only last for different lengths of time, but they are also sometimes gone through several times. These five phases are therefore only something like a rough orientation framework, the individual expression is different in reality for every person. They are something like a map, which should not be confused with the landscape.

Many also apply this five-stage model to the grief of the bereaved and for some this simple stage model of Kübler-Ross is now considered outdated, as it seemingly makes the grief for the relatives predictable (more on this see Chap. 10). Nevertheless, it is the framework that many hospice facilities orient themselves by.

According to other ideas, the grieving process of the bereaved is described as a tension field between two poles. On the one hand, there is the loss and grief for the deceased and on the other hand, there is the present and the future and the bereaved oscillate between these two poles of grief and hope back and forth.

Further Reading

Kübler-Ross, Elisabeth: Verstehen, was Sterbende sagen wollen, Stuttgart 1982 (Kreuz)
Kübler-Ross, Elisabeth (Hrsg.): Reif werden zum Tode, Stuttgart 1983 (Kreuz)
Kübler-Ross, Elisabeth: Was können wir noch tun? Stuttgart 1977 (Kreuz)
Schwikart, Georg: Die 100 wichtigsten Fragen zu Tod und Trauer, Gütersloh 2008 (Gütersloher Verlagshaus)

7

Jacob Levy Moreno (1889–1974): "Playing God" or Directing Until the Last Scene

Contents

7.1	Birth—Truth(s) and Poetry	61
7.2	Religious Influences	61
7.3	Name Changes	61
7.4	Religious Maturity	62
7.5	Working with Marginalized Groups	62
7.6	Sociometry	62
7.7	Literary Avant-Garde	63
7.8	Impromptu Theater	63
7.9	Emigration to the USA	64
7.10	From Impromptu Play to Psychodrama	64
7.11	Taking Responsibility with the Action Method	65
7.12	Psychodrama: Approaches	65
7.13	Psychodrama: Procedure	66
7.14	Psychodrama: Roles	66
7.15	Psychodrama: Techniques	67
7.16	Psychodrama: Precursors	69
7.17	Stabilization	69
7.18	Publications	69
7.19	Beacon Hill Sanatorium and Moreno Institute	69
7.20	International Recognition	70
7.21	Women and Family	70
7.22	Daily Routine and Personality	71
7.23	The Wise Elder	72

© The Author(s), under exclusive license to Springer-Verlag GmbH, DE, part of Springer Nature 2024
W. Gross, *As One Lives, So One Dies*, https://doi.org/10.1007/978-3-662-70061-7_7

7.24	Starvation?	73
7.25	Directing Until the Last Scene	75
7.26	Conclusion	77
Further Reading		77

> This chapter is about Jacob L. Moreno, who, compared to other psychotherapists, primarily sees himself as an artist and director. After a multifaceted and turbulent life, he feels his limits and sees his time has come to say goodbye. He goes to bed and simply stops eating. Even in this situation of constant weakness, he is the director of his own death. He consciously plays his role in the "drama of life" to the end, lets his students parade past his deathbed, and tries not to stand in the way of death and to accept it.

Everything ripe wants to die. Everything immature wants to live. Everything that suffers wants to live, to become ripe and cheerful and yearning for something further, brighter, higher. (Friedrich Nietzsche)

Overview

"Acting is more healing than talking" is the credo of a therapy method called Psychodrama. As a scientific method of Group Psychotherapy, Psychodrama was founded by Jacob L. Moreno.

There is hardly any psychotherapist of the first hour who brings as many different approaches, such a variety of ideas, and such great creative energy as Moreno. Until his death, he was probably the person who inspired the most theorists and practitioners to further develop group psychological work and social psychology.

Moreno not only developed Psychodrama, but he is also considered the founding father of group therapy in general, and he introduced sociometry, a series of diagnostic procedures for measuring relationships in a group—not to mention the countless books he wrote and journals he edited.

Jacob Levy Moreno was born on May 18, 1889, around 4 pm in the Romanian capital Bucharest as the first of six children of the Jewish-Sephardic merchant Moreno Nissim Levy and his wife Pauline. Pauline had been married to the man 18 years her senior when she was only 14 and is said to have been strongly mystically religious. Since her husband is often on business trips, she is more or less solely responsible for raising the children. She is not only the central reference person in the family during Jacob's early years, and he is probably her favorite son. Thus, the father is once again on the road at the birth of his firstborn.

7.1 Birth—Truth(s) and Poetry

And already here, myths and rumors surround Moreno's birth (and not only that), which he later also likes to fuel. For example, in his autobiography, he writes that he was born during a stormy night at dawn on a Sabbath day during a ship journey from the Bosporus to the Romanian city of Konstanza on a ship of unknown nationality. Moreno also chooses May 16, 1892, the commemoration day of the expulsion of the Jews from Spain, as his birthday in his self-definition. Therefore, Moreno's autobiographical information should probably be valued as "psychodramatic truths" and not taken at face value.

7.2 Religious Influences

From about 1893, Moreno, as a 4-year-old, attends the Sephardic Bible school ("Cheder") and learns to read the Old Testament in Hebrew. However, he is probably also so impressed by the Catholic influences of his mother and the rituals of the Greek Orthodox Church, which he experiences in a nearby basilica, that he breaks his right arm in an early psychodramatic "God game" when he is 5 years old.

In 1895, the family (probably fleeing from poverty and fear of pogroms) moves to Vienna. The father is also mostly on business trips in the Balkans from here. When Moreno starts attending primary school in Vienna in 1896, he initially rejects the first name Jacob (or "Jacques" as his mother calls him). Here begins a kind of self-concealment, which leads him to believe that he is a very special and unique creation of God. He believes he is on an extraordinary mission and (impressed by Jesus, Buddha, and Francis of Assisi) considers himself a kind of prophet from an early age. This also fits to his later handling of his own name:

7.3 Name Changes

Born as "Jacob Levy", he first takes his father's first name into his name in 1917—so for 10 years he calls himself Jacob Moreno Levy—and later makes the name Moreno his surname. From 1927 he calls himself "Jacob Levy Moreno", as he is known today. In this context, it should have played a role that in Hebrew "Moreno" is a title and means "our teacher".

7.4 Religious Maturity

From 1901, Moreno attends high school in Vienna and celebrates his "Bar Mitzvah" in 1902, which makes him religiously mature according to Jewish belief. When the family moves to Berlin in 1904, Moreno returns to Vienna alone after 3 weeks in Berlin as a 14-year-old, where he rents a room as a subtenant. In 1905, he drops out of high school, but later attends a Jewish school and studies philosophy first, then medicine from 1909. He partly finances his studies as a private tutor in wealthy families.

Together with Chaim Pessach Kellmer, he founds a "Religion of Encounter", which aims to help the needy directly. This also leads to the creation of the "House of Encounter", an asylum for refugees and immigrants.

7.5 Working with Marginalized Groups

Even during his medical studies, he was concerned with marginalized social groups. Thus, he worked with the prostitutes of Spittelberg in 1913 and 1914, who were considered contemptible sinners in Vienna at the time, and tried—supported by journalists—to establish a self-help group of prostitutes.

From 1915, he worked as a student "assistant doctor" in the Mitterndorf barracks camp, where he was supposed to be responsible for 12 barracks with 10 rooms each. Later, he worked for several months in the Sternberg war hospital in today's Czech Republic.

7.6 Sociometry

On February 5, 1917, he completed his medical studies and returned to the Mitterndorf refugee camp as a doctor after his promotion, where he primarily took care of the children's ward, but also general diseases and hygienic conditions. There, he also conducted his first sociometric experiments. His observations in this large group of people from various regions and cultures led Moreno to learn to perceive and analyze the social forces of attraction and repulsion within the group: A group is more than just the sum of its members for him. These experiences form the basis for his later work on sociometry, action research and the development of the method of psychodrama.

From 1918–1925, he worked as a factory doctor in the Vöslauer Kammgarnfabrik and as a community doctor in Vöslau (today: Bad Vöslau). It was during this time that Moreno gained a reputation as a "miracle doctor".

7.7 Literary Avant-Garde

Moreno's literary activity also began early (from 1908) (*The Realm of Children, Homo juvenis*). He moved like a fish in water among the various Viennese circles of artists, intellectuals, and philosophers who met for discussions in the various coffee houses: Arthur Schnitzler, Franz Werfel, Martin Buber, Peter Altenberg, Gustav and Alma Mahler were considered the avant-garde of the new culture. On the political level, many left-wing politicians were active in Vienna, which was then governed by the Social Democrats. The most famous of these was the Marxist Leo Trotsky. Moreno is also said to have met Alfred Adler during this time. A contact with Sigmund Freud, which is supposed to have taken place in 1912, is not documented. However, the Freudian Theodor Reik probably participated in impromptu games staged by Moreno from time to time.

Parallel to his medical work, Moreno wrote various books and texts, with the theme of God and divinity seeming to have captivated him: *The Deity as a Comedian, The Deity as an Author, The Deity as a Speaker*. But he also published other texts: *The Father's Testament, The King's Novel, Speech on the Moment, Speech on the Encounter…*

As Moreno belonged to various avant-garde artist circles in Vienna, he also became the founder and editor of the magazine *Daimon*, in which many artists published their texts. After just one year, he renamed the monthly magazine to *The New Daimon*.

7.8 Impromptu Theater

Last but not least, he also wrote psychological-theoretical texts—e.g. "The Impromptu Game". For as a teenager, Moreno was fascinated by impromptu theater. He admired the spontaneity and creativity of the children playing in the Viennese parks. From 1907, he developed a special form of impromptu games—initially with children. Much later, he staged his first public impromptu theater experiment titled "The Madhouse of the Lord of the World by Jakob Levy" at the Vienna Comedy House on April 1, 1921 at 10 p.m., which he later considered the actual beginning of the psychodramatic method.

With financial support from his brother, who had emigrated to the USA at an early stage, Moreno founded the impromptu theater in Maysedergasse, where impromptu games were played 2 to 3 times a week until 1924. In this "Theater of Spontaneity", later famous actors (such as Elisabeth Bergner and Peter Lorre) gained their first theater experiences with Moreno, which apparently were helpful for their later acting careers.

7.9 Emigration to the USA

Since 1921, Moreno had been considering emigrating to the USA—especially since his brother Wilhelm had been living in the United States for some time. In 1925, he traveled to the USA at the invitation of an electrical company. He had developed an electromagnetic image and sound recording process together with the brother of his then life partner, Franz Lörnitzo. However, after unsuccessfully offering the invention to the "General Phonograph Company" and the further development of this project finally failed, he turned to other topics and first of all learned proper English.

From then on, the United States became his central place of life. He initially lived in New York. However, since his residence permit was initially only temporary, he briefly traveled to Montreal in Canada to get a new residence permit for the United States, lived in various places in the USA, and then returned to New York in 1927, where he also received permission to practice as a doctor.

7.10 From Impromptu Play to Psychodrama

During this time, Moreno leads impromptu games ("Impromptu School") at the Plymouth Institute in New York, before founding his first private psychiatric practice and the "Moreno Laboratories Incorporation" in 1929. In January 1931, the first issue of his magazine *Impromptu* is published and he performs "Living Newspaper" in front of an audience, where current daily news is presented on stage.

Moreno's entire life is bursting with ideas, creative insights, and sitting with just one person to reflect would be far too boring for him. That's why he also says: "The two-dimensional couch of psychoanalysis is replaced by the three-dimensional space." Psychodrama is a group therapeutic method that was developed to give participants the opportunity to express their feelings in spontaneous and dramatic role-play.

Of great importance is to act out emotionally significant feelings that are related to personal problems. This is intended to achieve a "catharsis" and build new behavior. Current, past, or anticipated conflict situations are played out by the group members to express pent-up feelings. With the help of psychodrama, the group members should be supported in resolving their problems or seeing them from a different perspective and redefining them. The dramatic form practiced in this process is intended to facilitate the direct and immediate addressing of problems or conflicts. It is about experiences in action, not about recapitulation of words and thoughts.

7.11 Taking Responsibility with the Action Method

Moreno develops psychodrama as a special form of group psychotherapy, which he understood as an "action method". The goal is to activate the individual group members. They should take responsibility for themselves as individuals as well as for the group as a whole. Responsibility is not only seen as a matter of cognition in this action method, but as a provocation to action.

Group psychotherapy actively intervenes in rigid structures and tries to bring people trapped in rigidity to spontaneity and new creativity. Moreno himself went even further. For him, the goal of group psychotherapeutic and psychodramatic efforts was nothing less than a worldwide, creative revolution. Moreno believed that the achievements of the 19th and 20th centuries—namely the exploration of the unconscious, psychoanalysis, and depth psychology—must be supplemented by developing and exploiting the creative possibilities of humans to ensure the survival of humanity.

To understand what Moreno means by psychodrama and how psychodrama works, it is important to take a closer look at this method.

7.12 Psychodrama: Approaches

In addition to simple impromptu and role-playing, psychodrama distinguishes:

- **The therapeutic psychodrama:** Here, the entire process is unplanned (= experimental), the production is used as exploration and serves as a guideline for the continuation of therapy, everything plays "hic et nunc", in the here and now. The free association of psychoanalysis is replaced by free action.
- **The existential psychodrama** does not take place in the theater, but in the patient's real world.
- **In analytical psychodrama**, the analyst steps out of his observer role and participates in the performance.

In psychodrama, one acts associatively and spontaneously **acted** (for comparison: in psychoanalysis, verbalization is associative). Dreams are reenacted, traumatic situations are acted out, certain behaviors are practiced. The focus in psychodrama is on **acting out**.

In addition to the various psychodrama approaches, there are various offshoots: sociodrama, hypnodrama, behaviordrama, ethnodrama …

7.13 Psychodrama: Procedure

The classic psychodrama is divided into 3 phases in its procedure:

1. **Initial phase**: This phase is used to collect diagnostic material, reduce fears, defense mechanisms and resistances, and thus create a climate in which the group participants can act without fear. In this phase, the theme of the group crystallizes (or the protagonist is found). In addition, the scene is set up, and the roles are assigned.
2. **Action and play phase**: As soon as the scene is constellated, the main part—the action and play phase—begins. Situations are played through, past and future focus on the here and now of the psychodramatic scene. Reality of life takes shape on the psychodrama stage. The protagonist and the group experience the events in the game with an intensity that hardly differs from the real situation. The goal is the catharsis of the protagonist and the group.
3. **Conclusion and discussion phase**: Once the Psychodrama has been played out, the protagonist usually wakes up as if from a dream. The psychodramatic reality transforms back into everyday reality for him. Now each participant tells the protagonist what he felt and experienced during the game and how he perceived the Protagonist ("shared feelings" and "feedback"). This is followed by an analysis and interpretation—both by the therapist and by the other participants in the psychodrama.

This is followed by a **process analysis**, in which the process is viewed and analyzed from the meta-level.

7.14 Psychodrama: Roles

In the classic psychodrama, the following people appear:

- **Protagonist**: He is the main actor, who is found through one of the initial techniques (see Sect. 7.15) and who presents himself and his problems (according to the principle: individual therapy in the group).
- **Therapist**: He has 3 functions:
  - He promotes the dramatic actions of the protagonist (as "director"), and he leads him deeper into his emotions.
  - He sometimes actively intervenes in the psychodrama.
  - He interprets the events.

- **Assistant therapists** (Auxiliary Egos): They play certain roles that the protagonist needs for his presentation, and they help and reinforce the function of the therapist.
- **Audience**: Arises from the group situation (usually 5–10 people).

7.15 Psychodrama: Techniques

Although the most important element in psychodrama is the spontaneous play of scenes, Moreno and other psychodramatists have developed special techniques. Usually, the therapist/director suggests these techniques, always paying attention to whether they promote the therapy or training process of the psychodrama. However, they should only be used if they increase the possibilities for spontaneity, catharsis, and insight. There are no limits to the development of spontaneous techniques. Generally, the psychodramatic techniques that are applied can be divided into:

- **Initial techniques** ("empty chair", "psychodramatic vignette", "catathymic scene", etc.) aim to increase the emotional state of the individual group members and activate them for participation in the psychodrama.
- **Action techniques**: They help to advance the game, clarify situations, convert a verbal report into actions: "role reversal", "double", "high chair", etc. have a clarifying function. Other techniques like the "mirror" or "behind the back" are intended to confront the participant with his behavior.
- **Closing techniques** have the task of capturing emotional processes and evaluating their significance, drawing a balance and enabling outlooks on the future ("playback", "changing", "future projection").
- **Framework techniques** "provide a specific field within which the various action techniques can be used" ("magic shop").
- **Special techniques**: Only a selection will be presented here:
  - **Role reversal**: The protagonist and another group member exchange roles. In this process, the patient confronts himself. He experiences how he is perceived by others, what reactions his own behavior triggers, and how much it contributes to solidifying the conflict situation in which he finds himself.
  - **Monologue**: The protagonist speaks directly to the audience, giving spontaneous expression to his feeling. The authentic expression of the feeling is important. The suggestion to hold a monologue is correct when the protagonist cannot adequately express his feelings in the game. This technique is also suggested when the intensity of his

emotional involvement prevents him from continuing to work productively. The monologue then gives him the opportunity to distance himself from his own emotions and to consider which reactions have previously occurred in him.
- **Double**: This technique is used when the impression arises that the protagonist is being overwhelmed by the other people in the scene being played. It can also be incorporated into the process when the person in question obviously has difficulty expressing his true feelings. The director then assigns a helper ego to the protagonist, with this person standing behind the protagonist and acting simultaneously with him or for him. A great deal of empathy is required on the part of the helper ego, as it should develop a feeling for what the protagonist is currently experiencing. It often helps the protagonist just to have someone standing behind him, following his feelings and body movements.
- **Mirroring**: When it seems necessary for the protagonist to step back from his role for a while to see his role embodied in another person, this technique finds its meaningful application. Especially when the protagonist has great difficulty realizing how his behavior affects others. Through this technique, he becomes a listener and viewer, while a helper ego plays his role as similarly as possible, often with the instruction to the helper ego to deliberately distort the behavior of the protagonist.
- **Behind the back** ("behind the back"): The therapist asks the protagonist to give up the game and sit with his back to the other group members. These then discuss their impressions of him under the guidance of the therapist. This technique is intended—similar to the mirror image—to help the protagonist perceive how others see him and react to him.
- **Magic shop**: With the help of this method, the protagonist should be enabled to express his real goals and wishes. A group member or the director himself plays the owner of the magic shop, where no items are sold. What can be acquired there are mainly: values, personality traits or general wishes, such as strength, power, courage, success, quick-wittedness or possession. In order to get something, other valued characteristics or aspects of one's own person must be offered or exchanged. This offers the opportunity to find out what is really important to the person concerned, or to think about which characteristics of their own behavior are hindering them from achieving their own goals.

7.16 Psychodrama: Precursors

Certainly—Moreno developed psychodrama from improvisational theater as a scientific method that follows a specific methodology and has a therapeutic effect. However, there are naturally a multitude of precursors in the history of mankind:

The mystery plays of antiquity, the "Commedia dell'arte", **Reil's** "psychic cure method" and **Marquise de Sade's** theater performances at the beginning of the 19th century, which he staged with his co-patients during his asylum stay in Charenton, are considered precursors of psychodrama.

Let's return to the person of Moreno.

7.17 Stabilization

Moreno becomes a member of the "American Psychiatric Association" (APA) in 1931. From then on, his situation gradually stabilizes: He is the first to use the term "group psychotherapy" at an APA annual meeting and conducts sociometric studies in the Sing-Sing prison and at various state schools. His sociometric studies with prisoners and his work with girls in a reformatory receive strong resonance and make him known in the professional world. And these experiences also flow into one of his main works *Who shall survive?*.

7.18 Publications

In addition to the many book publications, the various series of writings and the various journal foundations, Moreno also produces 16-mm films from 1933 onwards and founds "Therapeutic Motion Pictures" in 1935—all with the aim of making his methods and views known. However, it takes quite a while—until 1953, that a psychodrama session led by Moreno is shown on US television.

7.19 Beacon Hill Sanatorium and Moreno Institute

In 1936, he settles in Beacon, 90 km north of New York City, where he lives on his property until his death. There he opens the "Beacon Hill Sanatorium" and the first psychodrama stage "Therapeutic Theatre for Psychodrama". In 1938, the "Psychodramatic Institute" is founded by him at the same location, of which he remains the director for a long time and which is renamed "Moreno Institute" in 1950.

7.20 International Recognition

Moreno developed Psychodrama as "the method that explores the truth of the soul through action", with the aim of "releasing human spontaneity and at the same time integrating it meaningfully into the entire fabric of human life".

The professional world's recognition of his method of psychodrama is long denied to Moreno. Only in the 1960s and 1970s does this therapy method receive more attention—under the motto: "Action is more healing than talking." By this time, Moreno is already well over 70 years old.

It is the three topics of "Sociometry", "Psychodrama" and "Group Psychotherapy" that are henceforth associated with the name Moreno. He is a lecturer at the Teachers College of Columbia University in New York, in Harvard and at other universities, organizes meetings of psychiatrists, psychologists and sociologists, founds societies ("American Society for Psychodrama and Group Psychotherapy", "American Sociometric Association") and initiates congresses. From the mid-1950s onwards, he is internationally active at many congresses (Switzerland, Spain, Israel, Italy, France, Argentina, Brazil, Japan…). And the honors increase: in 1969 he is awarded the golden doctorate diploma of the University of Vienna, he is honorary president of various group psychotherapy congresses over the years and receives an honorary certificate for his 50-year medical practice from the "Medical Society of New York" in 1966 and the doctor honoris causa from the University of Barcelona.

7.21 Women and Family

His relationship with the Catholic teacher Maria Viktoria Stefanie Lörnitzo ("Marianne"), who first becomes his medical assistant, then his "muse" and later his lover, begins in 1919. This relationship probably continues even when Moreno goes to the USA—at least for the first few years. Because in the first 5 US years, Moreno struggles a lot and is financially supported by his brother Wilhelm. He finally receives help from the child psychologist Beatrice Beecher, with whom a more intense relationship develops and whom he marries on May 31, 1928—also to get a permanent residence permit. When he announces his marriage to his Austrian lover Marianne Lörnitzo, it leads to the final break between the two.

The relationship with Beatrice only lasts 6 years and they mutually agree to divorce in 1934 when Moreno receives permanent US citizenship. From 1938-1948, he is married to Florence Bridge, with whom he has a daughter, Regina, born in 1939. In 1949, he marries the stage designer C. Zerka Toeman, with whom he remains until the end of his life. Their common son Jonathan David is born in 1952. Zerka Moreno becomes something like the executor of J. L. Moreno's estate.

7.22 Daily Routine and Personality

Dr. Gretel Leutz, who knew Jacob L. Moreno as a teacher in the last 20 years of his life, worked as an au pair for the Morenos in her youth. Later, she translated his standard work *The Foundations of Sociometry* and brought psychodrama back to Germany. She says about the person Moreno in an interview with me:

> **Interview**
>
> "He was extraordinarily vital, cheerful, warm-hearted. … This is especially evident in his dealings with children and mentally disturbed people. He had direct access to them, completely unobstructed by any role expectations. He could play with the children, he could laugh with the fools. I once saw him in the sanatorium speaking in some freely invented language with a patient who was otherwise mute, who otherwise did not speak at all, and he was saying bla, bla, bla, something like that, making such sounds, and the patient reacted immediately and in the end they laughed together, and he left.
>
> The important thing for me was that I lived in his house for a year at that time, because I was actually taking care of his daughter. And so I was in contact with him every day. Usually he got up around 8 o'clock in the morning, read his mail, and then we had our conversations.
>
> Then he liked to talk about Vienna, told me a lot about the time after the 1st World War. At that time he published a monthly magazine *The Daimon* and later in the 2nd year *The new Daimon*, together with Alfred Adler, Franz Werfel, Wassermann and others.
>
> He told me a lot about the Viennese milieu, the literary milieu. He wrote a lot of poetry during this time, and I myself was fascinated by poetry and literature at that time, and that was our common element.
>
> Around 10 o'clock he usually went to the sanatorium, worked with the patients, between 9 and 10 o'clock he made his rounds. … This was his private clinic. He had 25–30 seriously ill patients there. And in the afternoon he started writing. He usually wrote until 3 o'clock in the morning.
>
> I believe he rarely slept more than 5 hours, 4–5 hours. And yes, a few times a week in the afternoon he did Psychodrama with the patients, and always took me with him, because I wanted to study medicine, and that's where I learned the most from him. Also, what psychodrama can mean for dealing with these severely disturbed people."

7.23 The Wise Elder

Over time, Moreno becomes calmer and wiser. Gretel Leutz is astonished when she meets him again after a long time in Europe:

> **Interview**
>
> "I knew him for over 20 years. Of course, I didn't see him as often in the last years. I lived in Europe and only sporadically came to America. He was always the same to me.
>
> Of course, he got older, at the international psychodrama congress in Amsterdam in 1971 he seemed genuinely aged to me for the first time. This was expressed in a slowed-down speech. He had a different pose than he used to have. He used to dance around a lot and always had new ideas, was sparkling, and there his speech suddenly became more solemn…
>
> Well, he was always wise, but he used to enjoy clowning around. He sometimes seemed to me like the joker in a Shakespeare play. There in Amsterdam at this lecture, he was perhaps more, yes, perhaps like an old sage."

Moreno, described as vital, cheerful, and warm-hearted, usually works late into the night. In the morning he had visits with patients, from the afternoon he writes until the break of dawn. From 1973 he appears for the first time "sluggish". In this year—he is 84 years old—he arrives for the international congress for group psychotherapy. Gretel Leutz describes how she experienced him:

> **Interview**
>
> "Yes. In 1973 at the international congress in Zurich he was quite frail. He could hardly stand on his feet, even complained once that he felt so sluggish compared to before. But even there there were situations, hours, where he could suddenly tell stories about Vienna, as always, in the circle of friends.
>
> After this dinner, where Moreno was present, the board of the international society for group psychotherapy withdrew for a consultation, his wife went with them and I stayed, together with Mrs. Schindler, her daughter and maybe a few, two, three other people, with Moreno at the table. And probably it was the Viennese language of Mrs. Schindler that transported him back to his homeland, to his youth, and Moreno began to sparkle, he told about his literary encounters with Peter Lorre, told about Vienna, about his friendship with Peter Lorre and Peter Altenberger, about Franz Werfel, Max Brod, all the literati who carried the intellectual life of Vienna at that time."

When he returns from his European trip to the USA, something decisive has changed. Gretel Leutz:

> **Interview**
>
> "He is said to have been quite weak after his return to America. He still worked on his autobiography, but he was not doing well. However, an improvement is said to have occurred in early 1974, so that he could still go to an annual meeting of the clinical psychologists of the city of New York and even give a small lecture.
>
> He even went out to the café afterwards, and was once again his old self. But in March he fell out of bed one night—I don't know if he wanted to get up or what happened—he definitely had to be helped back. He probably had several small strokes. His speech was said to have been a bit slurred for a short time, but the next day he could speak again, although he was weak on his legs, which he had been for some time anyway. He had no clear signs of paralysis, that's for sure. But from that hour on, he ate nothing more!"

7.24 Starvation?

The fact that Moreno lies in bed and simply stops eating, of course, disturbs his entire environment. Everyone who knew him wonders what could be wrong with him and what could be the cause. Gretel Leutz says:

> **Interview**
>
> "When Mrs. Moreno informed me that Moreno was so frail and would probably die soon, and suggested to me whether I might want to come again, I asked her what was wrong with him, and Mrs. Moreno said: 'He is not eating anymore.' And I then suggested to her whether we could give him enzymes in a soup or something, and she said: 'No, he is not eating anything at all.' … I could not understand it. But when I sat by his bed and—I remember, we once talked about Vienna. … I did not know Vienna very well at the time, I had only been there once, but I mentioned a few places that I knew meant something to him. He gradually remembered. I then talked about Café Central, where he liked to go, about Café Mozart, and then he said: 'Yes, yes, those were the days.' And then I said: 'And the good Linzer Torte, right?' And he said: 'Yes, wonderful, and the nut crescents, yes delightful, and the cheese pancakes.' He was almost reveling. … Then I said to him: 'And how about we eat a little bit now?' And suddenly he made a very serious face and said: 'No.'
>
> I could imagine that he was certainly also without appetite, but undoubtedly he also had the feeling that his time was up, and he did not want to

> artificially prolong his life. He certainly experienced the loss of strength and his attitude was then 'let nature take its course', one must let nature run its course ...
>
> He was basically unchanged. He was bedridden, he could no longer get up, he only drank water. He could not talk for long, but he had short conversations, and when he had them, he was present. He was fully there.
>
> It was explained in such a way that everyone experienced that his time was coming to an end. And he did not want to artificially prolong it.
>
> His life was fulfilled, and he always had an intense relationship with death—in this volume of poetry *The Father's Testament* there is also a chapter 'My Death'—and he lay in anticipation of his death, and so it was. He was not depressed. He was not disturbed. He was waiting."

In April 1974—the group psychotherapy congress had begun in New York—Moreno had a series of minor strokes in Beacon (about 90 km from New York) that had weakened him. Gretel Leutz remembers:

> **Interview**
>
> "Yes, in the following days, old students and friends of his, colleagues who lived all over America, but came every year to this congress, visited him in Beacon. That is, I always announced them to Moreno, and he said: 'Yes, yes, he should just come.' And he then received these students individually, spoke a few words with them—actually trivial words—but very personal. 'How are the children, how is work? Is your dog still alive?' And these questions were answered. And there was a closeness to be felt.
>
> The conversations were very short—they were also exhausting for Moreno. When he could no longer, or—better said—before he could no longer, he then extended his hand to his visitor and said: 'I thank you for your visit, I wish you all the best.' The person in question shook his hand or kissed him or stroked him, depending on the relationship, and left the room. Rarely did anyone leave without tears in their eyes, or at least swallowing once. It was so everyday and in this everydayness absolutely extraordinary.
>
> So it seemed to me like an Old Testament event. It was something peculiar. For example, his student Dean Eleftery, who has spread psychodrama very widely in Europe, in Holland and also in the Scandinavian countries, came one day and I knew him quite well. He was with Moreno, came out and was quite angry with me. He said: 'What is going on here? This is criminal. You are letting him starve. Why don't you give him infusions?' I said to Dean: 'Yes, I said that on the first day too, but that's not possible.' ... And Eleftery was beside himself. He said: 'I will now speak to his son, I am going to New York, this is impossible!'
>
> Eleftery came back after 3 days, visited Moreno again, was longer than the first time—and also longer than many others—with him. And as he came out, he immediately headed towards me and said: 'It has to be this way. Nothing else can be done. This belongs to Moreno.'"

7.25 Directing Until the Last Scene

In this way, Moreno also directed this—his last—ceremony in a certain sense. Dr. Gretel Leutz:

> **Interview**
>
> "At that time, the 32nd annual meeting of the 'American Society of Group-Psychotherapy and Psychodrama', which Moreno had founded in 1942, took place in New York, and since the founding of this society, Moreno had given the opening speech every year. And in 1974, for the first time, he was unable to go. It was incredibly difficult for him, his wife Zerka went alone. I stayed with him at home, and when I was outside, the housekeeper called me, asking me to come, she could no longer keep Moreno in bed. I went into his bedroom—he already had one leg out of bed and wanted to get up, but he couldn't help himself and said to the housekeeper: 'I must go to the lecture.' He was driven, 'I must go to the lecture hall.' And then I spoke with him and said: 'Not all students who lived in Beacon at that time have gone to New York yet, some are still preparing sociograms, there's no rush.' I thought he might fall asleep again, but a quarter of an hour later Moreno was so driven again that it was clear to me: It was torture for him to stay in bed. And then I thought: Now I have to apply his own method, namely the reality test.
>
> I called the housekeeper and asked her to help me lift Moreno out of bed. He stood, I threw his robe over him, and we took two, three steps, on one side the housekeeper, on the other me, and he looked at me and said again, 'I must go to the lecture-hall'.
>
> And his gaze was as focused as ever, and at the same time he was looking at me. There was something, yes, his gaze was broken, smiling, knowing, it's not possible anymore. And we took three steps, then I said to him: 'You must be tired, don't you want to sit in the chair?'
>
> He sat in the chair and breathed heavily. And after some time we helped him back into bed, and it was clear to me: This must have been the bitterest situation of his life for this active, vital man. The will was still there, but now he could not realize it. He could not act. His method is an action method. He could not anymore. And then I remembered that I had brought his book *The Testament of the Father* with me, his poems, and I fetched these poems, which he had written around 1920, and I read him a poem, and I noticed how it resonated with him. He had his eyes closed.—He was all ears. And then I read him another one and another one. And after a while he had fallen asleep and I left.
>
> Later in the evening, Mrs. Schützenberger, his French student, returned from New York. She had been at the congress and told me that she couldn't stand it in New York anymore. She came with the words: 'Is he still alive?' And I said: 'Yes, yes, his condition is unchanged.' We sat there in a room upstairs together and talked for a long time, not only about Moreno. Suddenly the student, a black man who had been watching over him at night, came up and said, Moreno was speaking a language he no longer understood. He would also keep calling a name, so he couldn't cope with him anymore. Moreno insisted in this foreign language, and Mrs. Schützenberger immediately said to me:

> 'He can only mean you. Surely he is speaking German.' And then I went down to his death room with this student. A small lamp was burning, Moreno was awake. He recognized me. I asked what he wanted, and he only said, 'another poem' ... Then I read him another poem. Then there was a long pause, a long silence, because listening was also exhausting for him. After a while he woke up again, looked at me, 'another poem ...' Another poem. ... I will never forget this hour. There was a great closeness and yet Moreno was somehow already distant."

And yet it took a few more days until Moreno died. Gretel Leutz on his last days:

> **Interview**
>
> "Since the time I read him these poems, he spoke almost only German. And in the last days he is said to have spoken only German. His wife told me that on his day of death, or maybe the day before—I'm not sure—he said in the morning: 'Don't go to school!'
>
> It wasn't a school, but there were many psychodrama students in the sanatorium, whom Mrs. Moreno was teaching. And in German, the German word for school came to his mind ...
>
> He just got weaker and weaker. And in the last days he is said to have had a bowel bleeding and apparently once said to his wife: 'It was perhaps cancer after all.' But personally, I think, if an 85-year-old man has only consumed tap water for 6 weeks, no electrolyte, no vitamin, nothing at all, then it is not surprising that at some point the organs simply fail. Yes, that an artery might burst or that everything no longer works.
>
> And he is also said to have said very calmly on the last day: 'It is hard.' He accelerated this transition by not eating anymore. But Moreno was a person who loved life immensely, all his life. And I believe, that was hard for him.
>
> He never clung to life, but he always loved it, and he knew, now he is leaving this life. And that was hard for him.
>
> Zerka Moreno was with him shortly before, then away—for a short time of course. An old nurse, who had worked with Moreno for many years, was with him and sat by the bed when he fell asleep quietly."

On May 14, 1974, Moreno dies 4 days before his 85th birthday.

Moreno's mortal remains are transferred to Austria much later, where they are interred in an honorary grave in the urn grove of the Simmering crematorium on the Vienna Central Cemetery on September 6, 1993.

What Moreno had wished for many, many years ago as an inscription on his tombstone, happened. It says there:

"Jacob Levy Moreno, born 18.05.1889 (Bucharest)—died 14.05.1974 (Beacon/USA), founder of sociometry, group psychotherapy, psychodrama: 'The man who brought joy and laughter into psychiatry'".

7.26 Conclusion

Jacob Levy Moreno, compared to other psychotherapists, the artist, the actor, the clown, the director, sees his time as expired, goes to bed and simply stops eating (today it would be called "death fasting"). Even in the situation of permanent weakness, he is the director of his own death. He wants to consciously play out his role in the "drama of life", lets his students parade past his deathbed and tries—similar to some voodoo cults—not to stand in the way of death.

Further Reading

Engelke, Ernst: Psychodrama in der Praxis, München 1981 (Pfeiffer)
Erdmann, Z. M.: Psychodrama, Düsseldorf 1975
Leutz, Gretel: Das klassische Psychodrama nach J. L. Moreno, Heidelberg 1974
Moreno, J. L.: Die Grundlagen der Soziometrie, Köln/Opladen 1974
Moreno, J. L.: Gruppenpsychotherapie und Psychodrama, Stuttgart 1974
Petzold, Hilarion: Angewandtes Psychodrama, Paderborn 1978 (Junfermann)
Petzold, Hilarion: Psychodrama – die ganze Welt ist eine Bühne (aus: Wege zum Menschen, Bd. 1), Paderborn 1982 (Junfermann)
Schützenberger, Anne: Einführung in das Rollenspiel, Stuttgart 1976 (Klett)
Yablonsky, Lewis: Psychodrama, Stuttgart 1978 (Klett-Cotta)
Interview mit Dr. Gretel Leutz, direkte Schülerin von Jacob L. Moreno (1985)

8

Interlude IV: Types of Death and Styles of Dying

Contents

8.1	Definition and Transitions	80
8.2	Natural and Unnatural Causes of Death	80
8.3	Taboo Topic	81
8.4	Classification and Philosophical Interpretation	81
Further Reading		82

> This article discusses the different ways in which someone dies, i.e., their style of dying. It describes biological death as well as the handling of dying and death in different cultures. It explains the differences between natural and unnatural causes of death and the different terms we use for the dying of humans, animals, and plants.

Everyone wants to go to heaven,
but no one wants to die.

As a biological fact, death is something trivial. In death, laws are confirmed to which all of nature is subject: becoming and passing away, emerging, growing, reaching the peak, and then—the gradual—more or less rapid—descent, the decay, up to that qualitative leap. Speaking materialistically, one could say: Our energy is not lost, but it is absorbed in the biomass.

8.1 Definition and Transitions

Human death is clearly defined as a final state: when a person has lost relevant life functions, we speak of death—medically "Exitus". The dying process itself is referred to as the (intermediary) transition from life to death.

In this transition, the exact boundary between life and death is often difficult to define, as usually the organs do not all stop their activity at the same time. Since it is a process, the exact time of death is not easy to determine. Often, the reasons leading to death are multifactorial causes, i.e., several areas are damaged or disturbed. Organ failure, cardiac arrest, brain death are the central terms. In organ removal, "brain death" is considered a sure lethal sign.

Death is usually caused by failure of the cardiovascular system or the central nervous system (i.e., the brain and/or spinal cord). Among the reasons why people die, we distinguish between natural and unnatural causes of death. However, this distinction is not always clear-cut.

8.2 Natural and Unnatural Causes of Death

The **natural** causes of death mainly include diseases and the failure of body functions. Sometimes dying is hard work.

The **unnatural** causes of death are characterized by the fact that a severe injury is inflicted on the person from the outside—e.g., by an accident, a crime, a natural disaster, or war. Poisonings and suicides are also counted among the unnatural causes of death.

When trying to summarize the different types of death and styles of dying on a superficial level, the following categories can be formed:

- Death after a long illness,
- Result of a (wrong) lifestyle,
- Old age weakness,
- Sudden death (accident),
- Death by violent crime, war, pandemics etc.,
- Suicide: voluntary death or self-murder.

However, these are only the external descriptions—the inner, subjective perception of each individual can be experienced very differently. Because of course, every style of dying is as individual as a fingerprint: painful or relieving, struggling and resisting or without a fight, fast or slow, emotionally dramatic or quiet and silent.

8.3 Taboo Topic

Since death is still a taboo topic for many, there are more or less strange terms in almost all languages to describe death: "Grim Reaper", "Death's brother", "Sleep's brother", "Reaper". To depict the dying process, attempts are made to circumvent the finality of death with certain words and to emphasize the transition to another world: "to fall asleep", "to go home", "to pass away", "to fall" (e.g., in war), "to bless the temporal", "to embark on the last journey", "to perish". If it was a difficult type of death or inhumane circumstances during dying, people also speak of "croaking", "kicking the bucket", "biting the dust" or "scratching off". Animals, on the other hand, "die", are "put to sleep", "shot" by hunters. And plants "die off" or "wither".

One distinguishes regarding mortality between frequent and rare, but also between violent and non-violent causes of death. Not every disease that robs one of the joy of life leads directly to death: A wrong lifestyle can also be seen as an unconscious suicide in installments. Because the creeping causes of death also count: "The dose makes the poison", as Paracelsus already said. The mortality rates of the individual causes of death (cardiovascular diseases, cancer etc.) are not only distributed differently between men and women, old and young, rich and poor, but they are also very different in the various cultures.

8.4 Classification and Philosophical Interpretation

One thing is certain—death is the final end of the physical-organic and the active, physically detectable existence of a person. However, then comes the cultural, social and personal classification and philosophical interpretation, which can vary greatly:

- With death, everything is over. There is no (individual) soul that continues to live. Perhaps the energy is preserved and merges into the biomass etc.
- Death is only a phase for the person concerned, which eventually leads to a new individual life in this world (reincarnation).
- Death is the irreversible transition to another state of being (the soul is immortal, it continues to live in the realm of the dead, in the hereafter—or there is a resurrection at the Last Judgment). In any case, there is a (possibly eternal) life after death.
- In some mystical-religious schools (e.g. in Zen), they keep out: No statement is deliberately made about what happens after death.

Depending on how a culture deals with death, this has effects on the forms of burial and funeral rites, the tombstones and memorials, but also on the memorial dates and death customs. Whether the dead, like the Hindus, are mostly cremated, while this is not allowed for the Jews. Or whether the dead, as in Indonesia during the Ma'nene ceremony, are taken out of the graves and dried in the sun in their best clothes after a formaldehyde preservation, only shows how differently it is handled from culture to culture. And accordingly, there are very different ideas about what happens after death: Heaven, hell, purgatory, Last Judgment, limbo, rebirth, life after death etc. are the culturally and socially codified ideas according to which people live and die.

No matter how the individual culture, the own social reference group or one's self stands towards death and dying: A person is truly dead only when the memories of his or her person are forgotten.

Further Reading

Tausch-Flammer, Daniela, Bickel, Lis: Die letzten Tage, Stuttgart 1999 (Kreuz)
Heidepeter, Lothar Verbraucherzentrale: Was tun, wenn jemand stirbt? Berlin 2004
Wagner-Rau, Ulrike: Zeit mit Toten, Gütersloh 2015 (Gütersloher Verlagshaus)

9

Fritz Perls (1893–1970): "You Will Not Tell Me What to Do"

Contents

9.1	Education.	84
9.2	Exile.	85
9.3	Gestalt Therapy	85
9.4	Human Potential Movement	86
9.5	Image of Humanity	86
9.6	Philosophy.	87
9.7	Publications and Esalen	87
9.8	Restlessness and Impatience	88
9.9	Gestalt Prayer.	88
9.10	Awareness, Here and Now, and Growth	88
9.11	Freud and Perls.	89
9.12	Gestalt Therapy and Gestalt Psychology: Foundations	89
9.13	Sources of Gestalt Therapy.	90
9.14	Psychoanalysis	90
9.15	Gestalt Psychology	91
9.16	Behaviorism.	91
9.17	Psychodrama	92
9.18	Zen Buddhism.	92
9.19	Existentialism and Phenomenology	92
9.20	Wisdom of the Organism.	93
9.21	Practice	94
9.22	Gestalt Kibbutz	95
9.23	Restlessness	95

© The Author(s), under exclusive license to Springer-Verlag GmbH, DE, part of Springer Nature 2024
W. Gross, *As One Lives, So One Dies*, https://doi.org/10.1007/978-3-662-70061-7_9

9.24 Illness and Death 96
9.25 Dance of Death 96
9.26 Conclusion.. 97
Bibliography 97

> This chapter is about Fritz Perls, the central figure of humanistic psychology. He developed the Gestalt therapy as a method of psychotherapy. After a life full of ups and downs in various places around the world, Perls – it seems at least – would rather die than slowly succumb to rampant cancer. Throughout his life, he defiantly emphasized the "here and now" and his individual freedom. In the last minutes of his life, he does everything to prevent self-responsibility from being taken out of his hands. In the face of death, he essentially perishes out of resistance to the nurse's recommendations, who appeals to his reason, which he does not accept.

Lose your head and discover the meaning. (Fritz Perls)

> **Overview**
>
> Fritz Perls, who founded Gestalt therapy as a central method of humanistic psychology, was a peculiar person – in the double sense of the word "peculiar": On the one hand, he was an eccentric oddball who had developed many quirks and eccentricities in his directness – on the other hand, he was precisely because of this a person who in their uniqueness is **worthy** of being **remembered**.
>
> His life path is a single—more or less conscious search—full of errors and confusions, full of advances and setbacks.

Fritz Perls, the father of Gestalt therapy, was born as Friedrich Salomon Perls, on July 8, 1893, as the youngest of three children of the Jewish wine merchant Nathan Perls in Berlin. As a boy, he is said to have hated school, but he probably enjoyed acting in theater during his school years. Little is known about his early childhood.

9.1 Education

He studied medicine and served as a field doctor in World War I. He is also said to have been wounded. In 1921, he graduated as a doctor and began psychoanalysis with Karen Horney. From 1926, he was an assistant doctor to Kurt Goldstein, who introduced him to Gestalt psychology at that time. He completed his psychoanalytic training with Helene Deutsch and Otto Fenichel—later also with Wilhelm Reich, whom he was particularly impressed by and with whom he began a teaching analysis.

9.2 Exile

He had to interrupt his teaching analysis when the National Socialists took power in Germany in 1933. Like Reich, he also had to flee Germany. He first went to the Netherlands with his family and then to South Africa in 1934.

In 1936, Perls gave his first lecture titled "Oral Resistances" at a psychoanalytic congress in Czechoslovakia. This met with skepticism from most psychoanalysts and led to a first break with the orthodox psychoanalysts.

In 1941, Perls wrote his first book titled *The Ego, Hunger, and Aggression* together with his wife Laura, in which he already outlined the basic theoretical thoughts of Gestalt therapy. The subtitle also distinguishes it from psychoanalysis: "A revision of Freud's theory and method".

He emigrated to the USA in 1946.

9.3 Gestalt Therapy

Over time, Fritz Perls developed Gestalt therapy together with his wife Lore ("Laura") and with the collaboration of Paul Goodman.

Gestalt therapy is an experience-activating method of psychotherapy, in which the promotion of current awareness (Awareness), the perception of present feelings, sensations, and behaviors, and the contact with oneself and the world are in the foreground. Perls developed a typical experimental working method that quickly found followers.

His goal is unalienated life, in which spontaneity, emotionality, and contact with others are not distorted, twisted, or stunted. Authenticity is important to him: "Loose your head and come to your senses",—in the here and now. He revolts against any kind of dogmatism, is impatient, direct, provocative, and biting. He is offensive because he wants to initiate something. In doing so, he shows himself directly and openly. Freud's first biographer, Ernest Jones, not without reason called Perls an "exhibitionist".

9.4 Human Potential Movement

Thus, Perls is considered one of the most important founders and representatives of the "Human Potential Movement". This movement for the development of human potential and the humanistic psychology largely emerged as a counter-movement to the two established psychological directions in the USA – against **Behaviorism** and **Psychoanalysis**. Humanistic psychology therefore sees itself as the "third force" in psychology.

This third force developed mainly because many people had come to the conviction that both psychoanalysis and behaviorism unjustifiably foreground a pessimistic view of human nature. It is primarily the image of humanity of these two directions that displeases humanistic psychologists. Orthodox Freudians focus too much on animalistic drives—especially sexuality and aggression. The "higher" feelings are only seen as derivatives of the lower instincts.

Behaviorists, on the other hand, would view most mental processes only as psychological reactions to external stimuli. They would try to cure emotional disorders by conditioning behavior. Thus, both schools focused too much on pathological phenomena and paid too little attention to the normal and healthy.

Both theories—in the opinion of humanistic psychologists—care too little in their classical form about the central, optimistic characteristics that make humans human—and make an individual life worth living.

In contrast, humanistic psychology sees itself as a "psychology of optimism" and assumes that man is good at his core and that it is only a matter of bringing out the good in him.

9.5 Image of Humanity

Because humanistic psychology assumes that man is fundamentally good and healthy, it is only a matter of freeing this (buried by education, morality, environmental influences) good in him. Therefore, the loss of external control is initially good from the point of view of humanistic psychologists ("lose your head and discover the meaning"), just as any expression of emotions is seen as positive because it brings people closer to themselves, their true inner self ("becoming more oneself, more like, what one truly is").

The goal of Perls and the Human Potential Movement is therefore to help people achieve full emotional maturity and thus lead a fulfilled life according to their talents, character traits and preferences: the all-round developed, autonomous, healthy and natural person who is in harmony with himself, his emotions and needs and his environment. Perls writes:

"To be able to do that, there is only one way to go: become natural, learn to stand on your own, unfold your core and understand the basis of Existentialism. … I am what I am, and at this moment I simply cannot distinguish myself from what I am."

Thus, there are various terms in humanistic psychology, on which it is based: "Living in the here and now", "growth", "authenticity", "creativity", "joy" …

Perls writes: "Every individual, every animal, every plant has an innate goal—to realize itself, as it is."

9.6 Philosophy

Philosophically, the humanistic psychology is mainly based on existentialism and phenomenology (Buber, Heidegger, Husserl, Binswanger, Bühler), but is also influenced by Eastern philosophy, and by utopians like Aldous Huxley and George Orwell.

Its main philosopher Abraham Maslow tried to bring together like-minded philosophers and psychologists since the mid-1950s, until the Human Potential Movement emerged in the 1960s, whose most important method was and is Perls' Gestalt therapy.

9.7 Publications and Esalen

The book *Gestalt Therapy* was published in 1951. Perls wrote it together with Paul Goodman and Ralph F. Hefferline. In 1952, Fritz and Laura Perls founded the Gestalt Institute in New York, followed by another institute in Cleveland in 1953. From 1960 onwards, Perls dealt with existential psychiatry and got to know Zen Buddhism in Japan. In 1964, he landed at the Esalen Institute in Big Sur, California, the Mecca of the Human Potential Movement. Perls conducted his Gestalt therapy workshops with aspiring psychotherapists there. Through this—but also through films and book publications—Gestalt therapy became increasingly known in the USA and later also in Europe.

9.8 Restlessness and Impatience

Perls is driven in his life in a strange way and finds nowhere a real home—neither in Berlin, nor in Vienna, nor in South Africa, where he builds the "South African Institute for Psychoanalysis", nor in all the many places in the USA where he lives temporarily—and also not in Israel or Japan. And even later when he becomes one of the cult figures in the Esalen Institute, the Mecca of humanistic psychology, from the mid to late 1960s, this restlessness shows itself.

His lifestyle naturally also finds its reflection both in the theory and in the practice of Gestalt therapy.

Hilarion Petzold, co-founder of the German Fritz Perls Institute, believes that Perls, who was driven around all his life and could never settle down, therefore makes "the quiet serenity in the 'continuum of awareness' the core principle of his therapy".

Because the focus on awareness in the here and now relieves him of duration and obligation, because it emphasizes the encounter and neglects the relationship.

9.9 Gestalt Prayer

This is also evident in the "Gestalt Prayer" attributed to Perls:

> *I am I and you are you. I am not here to fulfill your expectations, and you are not here to fulfill my expectations. If we find each other, it's beautiful, if not, there's nothing to be done.*

This text (which, by the way, exists in various versions) is something like the open credo of Gestalt therapy—and also for the life of Perls.

9.10 Awareness, Here and Now, and Growth

Perls' emphasis on the Here and Now, the concept of Awareness, the role of direct encounter, the importance of personal Growth, all this is an expression of the personality of Fritz Perls, which is reflected in Gestalt therapy.

Hilarion Petzold considers Perls to be an advocate of the positive and constructive potential of aggression. This is also evident in the way he speaks and how he does therapy: "ad-gredi", directly approaching people and the world.

However, this directness is sometimes harsh, as it is an expression of the therapeutic concept of targeted frustration and direct communication. Thus, it is also an expression of the provocative, challenging, often also harsh nature of Fritz Perls.

9.11 Freud and Perls

Apart from the theoretical implications that distinguish Gestalt therapy from psychoanalysis, Perls' separation from psychoanalysis is certainly influenced by an earlier personal encounter with Freud, who receives him in Vienna in 1936 for a few minutes, fobs him off with an autograph and sends him away.

Perls never forgives Freud for this, and in his publications there are many jibes, malice and spitefulness against Freud and psychoanalysis. Not least because of this, many concepts of Gestalt therapy have been developed and formulated as antitheses to psychoanalysis. Perls writes:

"We do not need to dig à la Freud, down to the deepest unconscious. We must make the obvious conscious. If we understand the obvious, everything is there. Every neurotic is a person who does not see the obvious. So what we are trying to do in Gestalt therapy is to understand and see the word 'now', the present, the awareness of what is happening now." (Perls 1970, p. 25).

9.12 Gestalt Therapy and Gestalt Psychology: Foundations

The Gestalt Therapy combines the psychoanalytic conception of the unconscious and repression with insights from Gestalt psychology, which was founded as a counter-current to the "elementaristic" conception of the first experimental psychologists around Wilhelm Wundt by Wertheimer, Köhler and Koffka.

The Gestalt Psychology begins to play an important role after the emigration of its leading representatives to the United States. It has confirmed its reputation in Gestalt therapy of providing valuable practical suggestions, stimulating original experiments (like those of Kurt Lewin, who founded the scientific Group Dynamics), but not providing a systematic theory, as psychoanalysis attempts.

9.13 Sources of Gestalt Therapy

In addition to **Psychoanalysis**, the following psychological and philosophical methods are considered further sources of Gestalt therapy:

- Gestalt psychology,
- Psychodrama,
- Behaviorism,
- Zen Buddhism,
- Existentialism and Phenomenology.

9.14 Psychoanalysis

The most significant differences between the Gestalt approach and psychoanalysis are:

- the phenomenological versus the causal view of psychoanalysis,
- the focus on the present versus the (psychoanalytic) focus on the past,
- the principle of Gestalt dynamics (i.e., the emergence, closure, and integration of psychological Gestalts) as opposed to the libido principle,
- the assimilation of emotions as opposed to the discharge of emotions,
- the client's self-interpretation as opposed to the external interpretation of psychoanalysis,
- the close, intensive interaction of the therapist, who also reveals himself as a human being, as opposed to the distancing (mirror) attitude of the psychoanalyst. ("Freud invented the couch because he couldn't look people in the eye." [Perls]).

Perls' detachment from psychoanalysis began as early as 1936 with his lecture "The Dynamics of Oral Resistance".
 He criticizes psychoanalysis for:

- treating psychological facts in isolation from the organism (similar to Reich),
- making a linear associative psychology the basis for a four-dimensional system,
- neglecting the problem of differentiation.

Perls' alternatives are:

- to replace the psychological concept with an organismic one,
- to replace associative psychology with Gestalt psychology, and
- to apply differential thinking (S. Friedländer's "creative indifference").

9.15 Gestalt Psychology

From the Gestalt psychology of the Berlin School (Wertheimer, Koffka, Köhler, Lewin), Perls adopted the "figure-ground phenomenon" and the "Gestalt psychological organization laws" (laws of the "good Gestalt", the "good continuity", the "proximity", the "Gestalt closure" and the law of "balance").

The term "Gestalt" means something like wholeness, entirety. Gestalt psychologists say that all human behavior, all human experience is based on "Gestalts" (basic principles, patterns).

According to Gestalt psychology, "the whole is more than the sum of its parts". According to Perls, all experience—not just visual—is summarized into such "Gestalts". We perceive the entire world—the world within us and the environment outside of us—as a meaningful whole and not as a series of unrelated stimuli.

The goal of Gestalt therapy is thus to close "unfinished Gestalts" ("unfinished business", unfinished situations, unresolved matters).

9.16 Behaviorism

Although humanistic psychology vehemently distances itself from Behaviorism on the one hand, on the other hand, Perls himself has described the Gestalt approach as "behavioristic phenomenology". He adopts the "stimulus-response model" from behaviorism, but processes it in a non-behavioristic way:

"The great thing about the behaviorists is that they actually work in the here and now. They look, they observe what is happening. If we could subtract the compulsion to condition from today's American psychologists and simply keep them as observers: If they could realize that the changes that are required cannot be achieved by conditioning, that conditioning always produces artifacts and that the real changes occur in other ways." (Perls 1974, p. 67)

This means that Perls does not accept the particularly strong external control of the patient by the behaviorists, nor the omnipotence of the therapist (who godlike creates the right conditioning programs) and of course cannot approve of the total planning and the absence of any spontaneity.

9.17 Psychodrama

Another psychological direction on which Gestalt therapy is based is the Psychodrama developed by J. L. Moreno. A large part of the treatment techniques in Gestalt therapy are adopted from this (role play, role exchange, acting out of thoughts and dreams).

However, the bulk of the Gestalt dramas take place within the client. Stages, scaffolding, or scenes are very rarely set up; they mostly take place within the client, with the client assigning roles to certain feelings, as they are currently present in the body or in the thoughts, and playing them out.

In addition, the concept of "here and now" (one of the central terms of Gestalt therapy) is borrowed from Moreno.

In Gestalt therapy, it is assumed that all "unfinished Gestalts" reproduce at every moment—here and now—and can be consciously experienced in the present, with a strong focus on the "what" (content) and the "how" (behavior, focus of perception, existing emotional strength etc.), while the "why" (the focus of psychoanalysis) is put in the background.

9.18 Zen Buddhism

From Zen Buddhism, Perls mainly adopts "the awake attention in the now" ("awareness in the now") and the "beginner's mind".

9.19 Existentialism and Phenomenology

The Gestalt approach, however, is not only understood as psychological therapy, but also as an attitude towards life and philosophy of life.

"Gestalt therapy is a philosophy that wants to be in harmony, that wants to be in accordance with everything, with medicine, with the natural sciences, with the universe, with everything that is." (Perls 1974, p. 25).

In other places, Perls refers to "Gestalt" as "therapeutic philosophy" or "philosophical therapy". Thus, in his "Gestalt kibbutz" founded in

Vancouver, B. C., at the end of the 1960s, the differences between philosophers, psychotherapists, and educators should completely disappear—all according to the ideal of the "completely self-unfolding and self-determining human being" that no professional group restricts.

In addition to Binswanger's Daseinsanalysis and Frankl's Logotherapy, the Gestalt approach is the third therapy based on phenomenological Existentialism.

The philosophical background is mainly provided by the various theories of existentialism, especially those of Husserl, Buber, Heidegger, Friedländer, and Sartre.

9.20 Wisdom of the Organism

According to this idealistic view of Perls, we can rely on the wisdom of the organism. For the opposite of this is the disease of self-manipulation, which disrupts this finely tuned organismic self-rule.

Mental illness is accordingly seen as a disturbance of this dynamic process, with the avoidance of important "figures" at the center. Crucially important parts of the self—desires, thoughts, feelings—are avoided or actively excluded from conscious perception because they cause pain and/or fear.

Because no figures are formed here and thus no possibilities of satisfaction are sought, these areas cannot be integrated into the personality and overcome. They limit the activities of the individual and deprive him of energy, which is constantly tied up in these "unfinished tasks".

At this point, the dimension of here and now becomes convincingly apparent. If the organism is enabled to live as it wishes to live here and now, not towards the future or still bound in the past, then it is completely itself—satisfied and healthy.

The inability to live in the here and now (always fleeing into fantasies, wishful dreams, fears) is therefore already seen at least as a precursor to illness.

Perls writes: "Awareness per se can already be healing; for through full awareness one comes into contact with the organismic self-regulation. One can let the organism take over the steering, without intervening oneself or interrupting its function."

The main goal of Gestalt therapy is for the individual to learn to stand on his own feet and take responsibility for himself and his life, to become aware of himself and thus to shape his life more satisfactorily himself. This is certainly a high and idealistic claim.

Gestalt therapy offers an approach as individual and group psychotherapy, in which the patient enters into an intense dialogue with himself. He gives expression to feelings, conflicts and prejudices of the immediate moment. Even from the purely technical aspects, a demarcation from psychoanalysis and its very intellectual, discursive and past-oriented dialogue between analyst and patient becomes visible. Instead, action directed towards immediate experience is realized.

Perls writes: "We do not dig in an area about which we know nothing, in the so-called unconscious. I do not believe in repression. The whole theory of repression is wrong. We cannot repress a need. We have only repressed certain expressions of these needs. We have blocked one side, and then the self-expression comes out elsewhere, in our movements, in our posture and especially in our voice. … The pressing unfinished situations come to the surface in any case. We do not need to dig: It is all there." (Perls 1974, p. 31).

Gestalt therapists therefore assume that the repressions (Gestalt: unfinished situations) of the physical and mental needs of humans express themselves in the **here and now**, can be perceived and can also be therapeutically processed.

9.21 Practice

In Gestalt therapy, work is therefore done on 3 levels:

1. Externally recognizable behavior (actions, gestures, facial expressions, body posture, speech modulation, etc.).
2. Physical sensation of the patient, which he should communicate.
3. Mental activities taking place in the patient ("where is your attention?").

The focus is much more on the "what" and the "how" than on the "why".

The question of "why" is seen by Perls as rationalization, as a waste of time, as mental masturbation ("mind-fucking").

"When you ask **how**, you look at the structure, you see what is happening now, you have a deeper understanding of what is happening. The **how** is all we need to understand how we or the world function. The **how** gives us perspective and orientation. The **how** shows the validity of one of the basic laws, namely the identity of structure and function. … **Now** encompasses everything that exists. The past is no more, the future is not yet. **Now** includes the balance of being here, is experience, engagement, phenomenon, awareness. … I know, you want to ask **why** – like every child, like every immature person asks **why** to have rationalization or an explanation. But the **why** leads at best to a clever explanation, but never to an understanding. **Why** and **because** are evil words in Gestalt therapy. The **why** only results in an incessant questioning of the reason for the reason for the reason for the reason." *(Perls, 1974, p.51/52).*

9.22 Gestalt Kibbutz

After Perls became the "guru" of the "Human Potential Movement" at the Esalen Institute in California in the 1960s, he decided to found a "Gestalt Kibbutz" as a working and living community at Cowichan Lake in Canada. The kibbutz aimed to go beyond a mere therapeutic objective and provide a space for personal growth.

According to Perls, people should develop there who are more than just "psychotechnicians". The nonsensical separation between philosophers, therapists, and educators for Perls should be overcome in their life and work. For Perls, Gestalt is not a technique, not a quick therapeutic method, but a serious way to find and grow oneself.

This growth is a process that takes time. According to Perls, Gestalt therapy requires an attitude that is not acquired in 2 months, but through long and serious training, at the center of which is the development of one's own personality.

He later described this brief year that he lived in Cowichan as the happiest time of his life.

9.23 Restlessness

But by the end of 1969, he is seized by restlessness again. Quite unexpectedly, he embarks on a solo trip to Europe, where—according to his wife Laura—he aimlessly moves from one city to another, from one theater to another, from one opera to the next.

He was already very ill at that time. When he returned to the USA in early 1970, his physical condition worsened considerably—he was in great pain.

9.24 Illness and Death

When he asks a friend who is a doctor for a diagnosis, he is told quite openly: pancreatic cancer. After an examination in a hospital in Chicago, he is artificially fed because he is getting weaker and weaker. Due to the severe pain, he is given anesthetics. After a long and difficult, 3-hour operation, he lies on his hospital bed connected to many tubes and wires.

He clearly tells his doctor that he would rather choose death than continue living with a proliferating cancer. He repeatedly demands that the infusion tubes and wires, which made him feel chained to the bed, be removed. When the nurse tries to calm him down, he becomes increasingly agitated and tries to get up. She calls the head nurse and she tells him, who already has his legs out of the bed again, that he must lie down again. He looks at her and says to her: "You will not tell me what to do." Then he collapses and dies.

It is March 14, 1970, around 8:30 pm when Fritz Perls dies of a heart attack, shortly before his 77th birthday. The autopsy reveals that he really suffered from a deep-seated pancreatic cancer. Perls preferred to die rather than give up his self-assertion and self-responsibility.

9.25 Dance of Death

He had previously announced that he wanted to be cremated, and that dance therapist Anna Halprin should dance with the guests for him at his funeral. Thus, 1200 people danced a sacred dance from the Jewish tradition in the San Francisco Civic Auditorium by candlelight, which is about the worship of God and the celebration of life and death.

His wife Laura (or: Lore) Perls continues to work in Gestalt therapy after his death and tries to continue their common legacy. She continues to lead training, further education, and supervision groups until 1989 and continues to work as a teaching therapist and mentor.

Due to her deteriorating health, she returns to her birthplace Pforzheim in May 1990, where she dies on July 13, 1990. Her urn is buried together with that of Fritz Perls in the Jewish cemetery in Pforzheim, where the couple's common grave is still located today.

9.26 Conclusion

Fritz Perls, the "guru" of humanistic psychology, seems to prefer to die rather than slowly perish from a proliferating cancer. He, who emphasized his "here and now" and his individual freedom almost defiantly throughout his life, does everything to ensure that his self-responsibility is not broken. His demand for direct communication turns in the face of death into the demand for direct action. This fits both his personality structure and the Gestalt therapy he developed. He dies, as it were, in resistance to the "reasonable" orders of the nurse.

Bibliography

Gaines, Jack: Fritz Perls – Here and now, Millbrae, California 1979 (Celestial Arts)
Kempler, W.: Grundzüge der Gestaltfamilientherapie, Stuttgart 1975
Passons, W. R.: Gestalt Approaches in Counseling, New York 1975
Perls, F. S./Hefferline, R. F./Goodman, P.: Gestalt therapy, New York, Julian Press 1951
Perls, Friedrich, S.: Gestalt, Wachstum, Integration, Paderborn 1980 (Junfermann)
Perls, Friedrich, S.: Gestalt-Wahrnehmung, Frankfurt 1981 (Verl. Hum. Psychologie)
Perls, Friedrich,S.: Gestalt-Therapie in Aktion, Stuttgart 1974 (Klett)
Perls, Friedrich, S.: Grundlagen der Gestalttherapie, München 1970 (Pfeiffer)
Petzold, H.: Gestalt-Therapie und Psychodrama, Kassel 1973 (Nicol)
Polster, Erving u. Miriam: Gestalttherapie, München 1975
Resnik, Stella: Gestalt-Therapie, in: Psychologie heute, Februar 1975
Ruitenbeek, Hendrik M.: Die neuen Gruppentherapien, Stuttgart 1974

10

Interlude V: Grief and Humor

Contents

10.1	Grief is not a Disease	100
10.2	Stages of Grief	100
10.3	Numbness and Stupor:	101
10.4	Sadness and Longing:	101
10.5	Disorganisation, Searching and Separation	102
10.6	New Orientation and Recovery	102
10.7	Laughing Tears: Grief and Humor	103
10.8	Humor as a Coping Strategy	103
10.9	Humor and Cynicism	104
Further Reading		105

> This article is about grief and the feelings associated with it. It describes the various stages of grief, as well as the importance of an appropriate grief response for healing. It also explains the strange connection between grief and humor—because humor can be a therapeutic tool, especially in the difficult times of grief.

It's not about how long we live, but how intensely and deeply we live.

Grief can be understood as a normal reaction to an abnormal situation, when one has lost someone (or something) that is important. This could be the severe loss of a loved one (death or separation) or a revered person, but also the loss of a job. However, grief can also arise from significant changes in life, such as a chronic illness or the limitation of a biological or physical function (e.g., sexual disorders, disabilities). It can also be triggered by an ideal loss or the memory of such losses: all the missed opportunities and/or the unlived life that one has left behind. Suddenly one becomes aware of how much lifetime one has wasted or squandered.

Grief is almost always accompanied by intense depression, hopelessness, lack of desire and joy, painful feelings, lack of courage, and depressive moods. And it can be associated with a whole range of unpleasant feelings: despair, anger, pain or numbness, linked with a "leaden heaviness". Feelings of meaninglessness can occur and last for varying lengths of time.

However, how an individual experiences and expresses grief also depends crucially on the culture and social environment. Sometimes grief is also religiously influenced—namely by the (more or less conscious) violation of explicit or implicit norms of the (religious) community. And this is often associated with feelings of guilt, self-doubt, and self-reproach.

10.1 Grief is not a Disease

Grief is not initially a pathological disorder and to alleviate it, compassionate and partnership conversations can sometimes help the affected person at first. However, if a grief reaction persists for a very long time after the triggering event and/or the stress level significantly deviates from normal grief, a disorder requiring treatment can develop. The distinction between a normal grief reaction and a pathological development, i.e., an abnormal loss reaction, depends on the duration of the grieving period and the type of grief reaction. The affected individuals then do not reach the phase of adjustment and reorganization, because in the case of excessive grief reactions, the person concerned is unable to go through the various phases of a normal grieving process.

10.2 Stages of Grief

Especially in people who have lost a loved one, it is often seen that they go through various stages of grief—even if they sometimes oscillate between the individual stages. Here are the typical stages of grief:

10.3 Numbness and Stupor:

In the first phase, the affected individuals do not want or cannot acknowledge the loss. They feel unable to perceive and accept the news (e.g., of death or separation). Typical statements are: "I simply can't grasp it", "That's impossible", "That can't have happened" or "It seems totally unreal to me". The affected individuals emotionally shut themselves off. The emotional isolation and denial is also a way to give themselves more time to process the loss. In this phase, the affected individuals appear petrified and emotionless and are in a "state of endurance" or "shock paralysis". The routines are initially continued as if in a trance.

This stage of grief is usually short. It lasts only a few hours or days. However, there is a constant tension—often associated with feelings of fear. The external (apparent) calm can be replaced within fractions of a second by an outbreak of intense emotions (crying, whimpering, screaming).

10.4 Sadness and Longing:

Gradually, the individuals become aware of the gap created by the loss of the partner. Because the future they had imagined is no longer possible. In this phase of grief, the affected individuals initially seek comfort in the memories of the person who is now no longer there, and try to be close to them by filling the void with idealized memories. As soon as the individuals have faced reality, intense emotions such as grief, pain, fear, frustration, feelings of guilt, and anger break through. This anger can be directed at "fate" ("why does this have to happen to me"), at oneself, at other people, or even at the person who is no longer there. Cognitively, the individual knows that they cannot blame her—but on an emotional level, they are still angry. Often, they then feel guilty because they are now also angry at the person they love. This phase is characterized by the breaking out of chaotic emotions, which occur after hours or days. Now the pain of grief breaks out unfiltered and is intensely experienced. The emotional state oscillates back and forth between grief, fear, and anger, between helplessness, self-pity, and feelings of guilt. Restlessness, "being under tension" and sleep disorders often accompany this. Sometimes the affected individuals then also embark on the aforementioned search for culprits. Sometimes there is weight loss or gain, alcohol or other substance abuse. There can also be unpredictable outbreaks of unfounded cheerfulness, where everything seems to be forgotten.

10.5 Disorganisation, Searching and Separation

Gradually, the person concerned becomes aware of what the loss really means. He/she slowly consciously accepts what has really changed for him/her. Now depressive symptoms become more openly apparent. Often there is apathy, persistent sadness, loneliness, disinterest and aimlessness, perhaps even physical weakness. A feeling of hopelessness spreads, as if life could never get better again and as if life without the deceased no longer makes sense. At the same time, however, there are also initial opposing impulses to free oneself from memories. Gradually, the person concerned is torn between the idealization of the departed person and the care of the mementos on the one hand, and the desire to get rid of and throw away all the past on the other hand. The same ambivalence also applies between seeking out and avoiding places that remind one of the deceased person. The goal in this phase is to accept that the loss is permanent and the search for the deceased is ended. If this phase is not overcome, life continues to be dominated by grief and depression. The feeling of life then has a lasting negative and hopeless tone.

10.6 New Orientation and Recovery

In this final phase of grief, faith in life gradually returns. Now the reality of the loss is fully accepted. At the same time, hope is regained.

After accepting the loss, the mourner takes on new tasks and roles again. Habits are reorganized. New goals are set and new relationships are started: The affected person approaches people again. The old strengths are rediscovered. The person concerned can laugh again and begins to develop again. The realization that life can be positive even after the loss takes hold. The (self-) confidence slowly returns. The grief is not completely gone, but the loss recedes more and more into the background. The pain decreases, but it only disappears completely after a longer period of time.

To avoid any misconceptions—these phases do not proceed schematically nor do they apply to all people in the same way. Each person goes individually through their own grieving process, which can differ significantly from other people. What can be said, however, is that grief wants to be suffered and endured in order to make itself superfluous. Repression, on the other hand, blocks and freezing kills the feelings. Each person deals with the loss of a loved one in a different way, but grief is a necessary process in the face of a loss. If one understands one's feelings, is supported by close people and takes care of oneself, one can overcome grief—and later even recognize how important it was for the person(s) affected.

10.7 Laughing Tears: Grief and Humor

Life does not stop being funny when people die. Likewise, it remains serious when people laugh. (George Bernard Shaw)

"The living close the eyes of the dead—the dead open the eyes of the living," says a Slavic proverb. The relatives of a deceased person have to live with the death of the deceased. And that is certainly not easy. But do we have to make it even harder for ourselves through the prescribed solemn mourning rituals than it already is? Unspoken, sad faces are demanded at funerals, everything is subdued, slow and heavy—especially in Central Europe. The different death rites in the various world regions can be well observed in the Kassel "Museum for Sepulchral Culture".

Often it is on the individual level like this: Those who have lost an important person sometimes hardly dare to laugh anymore. Yet humor can be extremely liberating: It can be a break from pain, making suffering bearable at least for a short time.

The involuntary bursting out, embarrassing laughter in the church or at the funeral is something like a pressure relief valve—similar to the excessive alcohol consumption during a "funeral feast", which loosens the tongue and tries to shed the heaviness of grief.

10.8 Humor as a Coping Strategy

In this context, humor—especially for mourners—can be a coping strategy. "Humor is when you laugh anyway," says a German proverb, and the American writer William Saroyan wrote: "With humor, it's like with oysters: A pearl presupposes a small wound."

So one can also say that the training to be a survivor is all too often associated with many emotional pains that are not easy to bear. And humor can sometimes help—because it can also be a protective factor. Often humor is linked with wisdom and can therefore help to achieve lightness. When someone says: "My expiration date has expired" or a cancer patient has set "Play me the song of death" as a cell phone ringtone, these are signs of a certain ironic distance to their difficult situation—which is often helpful in itself.

10.9 Humor and Cynicism

However, it is important not to confuse humor with cynicism and sarcasm and, even worse, to use it as a weapon against those who are grieving. After all, there are many different types of humor: conciliatory and compassionate humor, self-irony, gallows humor, black humor …

One thing is clear: good humor requires courage: "Where the fun ends, humor begins," a wise person once said. Because humor turns many things upside down and is a kind of key to the soul. The Austrian father of logotherapy, Victor Frankl, wrote: "Nothing allows the patient to distance himself more from himself than humor."

In his book *At the End, It's Not Over with Fun—Humor in the Face of Dying and Death*, Harald-Alexander Korp has compiled a whole series of experiences to better cope with our own finiteness and that of our relatives. He describes what humor is, how it works, and how it helps to better cope with dying and death. This ranges from the description of individual fates, through a "humor anamnesis" and striking aphorisms to pitch-black jokes:

- When the doctor says to the patient, "You are terminally ill," the patient asks desperately, "How much longer?" The doctor says, "Ten." The patient despairs, "Ten what? Years, weeks, days?" The doctor: "Nine, eight, seven…"
- "Humor despite (defies) tumor."
- "No thank you, we're not dying," says the housewife when death is at the front door.
- "Clear above and tight below, dear God, I want nothing more."

But of course, there are also many other aphorisms that take a humorous view of dying and death:

- When you're in the coffin, they've fooled you for the last time.
- The cemeteries are full of people who thought they were irreplaceable.
- Training for the dance of death: Sports and gymnastics fill graves and urns.
- "Anti-aging really makes no sense for you."

- "You were at Peter's funeral?" "Yes, but he wasn't very popular. I was the only one who clapped."
- In the end, every life is rewarded—or punished—with death.
- "Immortality is not everyone's cup of tea," Goethe is said to have said.
- Only one letter distinguishes between a malicious humor and a malignant tumor.

Each of us survivors still has a meaningful life ahead of us—how long it will last, no one knows. What it will look like, no one knows either, but we can take it into our own hands. Because humor is an attitude towards life—everyone has it or can develop it.

Further Reading

Hurzlmeier, Rudi (Hrsg.): Sensenmann, Oldenburg 2011 (Lappan)
Korp, Harald-Alexander: Am Ende ist nicht Schluss mit lustig, Gütersloh 2014 (Gütersloher Verlagshaus)
Mauss, Hans-Jörg: Fröhlicher Friedhof, Hamburg 2014 (Förderkreis Ohlsdorfer Friedhof)
Meidinger-Geise (Hrsg.): Komm, süsser Tod, Freiburg/Heidelberg 1982 (Kerle)
Pisarski, Waldemar: Anders trauern, anders leben, München 1982 (KaiserTB)
Simhandl, Christian, Mitterwachauer, Klaudia: Depression und Manie, Wien 2007 (Springer)
Sonntag, Martin (Hrsg.): Auf Leben und Tod, Oldenburg/Hamburg 2016 (Lappan)
Spiegel-Rössing, Ina, Petzold, Hilarion: Die Begleitung Sterbender – Theorie und Praxis der Thanatotherapie, Paderborn 1984 (Junfermann)
Wolfersdorf, Manfred: Depression, Berlin/Heidelberg 1994 (Springer)

11

Carl Gustav Jung (1875–1961): Anticipation of the Coming Adventure

Contents

11.1	Personality No. 1 and No. 2	109
11.2	Mother	110
11.3	Father	110
11.4	Family	110
11.5	Faints	111
11.6	High School	111
11.7	Studies	111
11.8	Burghölzli	112
11.9	Dissertation	112
11.10	Starting a Family	113
11.11	Jung's Relationship with Freud	113
11.12	Points of Contention	114
11.13	Analytical Psychology	115
11.14	The Scandalous Affair: Sabina Spielrein	115
11.15	Toni Wolff	116
11.16	Private Practice and Travels	116
11.17	The Reputation Rises	116
11.18	National Socialism	116
11.19	Honesty and Humility	117
11.20	Near-Death Experiences	118
11.21	Suffering Success	118
11.22	Death of the Wife	119
11.23	Preparations for Dying	120
11.24	Initial Dreams	120

© The Author(s), under exclusive license to Springer-Verlag GmbH, DE, part of Springer Nature 2024
W. Gross, *As One Lives, So One Dies*, https://doi.org/10.1007/978-3-662-70061-7_11

11.25	Death Wedding Procession.	121
11.26	Saying Goodbye.	121
11.27	"How wonderful …"	122
11.28	Hour of Death.	122
11.29	Synchronicity and Reincarnation	122
11.30	Funeral.	123
11.31	Conclusion.	124
Bibliography.		124

Trailer

This chapter is about the mystically oriented psychotherapist Carl Gustav Jung. This visionary engaged with the supernatural and the unexplainable from an early age. This is also reflected in the analytical psychology he developed. Death and dying were also early topics for him. Essentially, he prepared for his death for many years of his life after his first heart attack. At the moment of dying, he is repeatedly surprised that he is still conscious. Jung faces death prepared, curious about a new adventure, for him death is not the end. Does the human being dissolve in his "shadow" at the moment of his death? In the end, all that remains for him are the words: "How wonderful".

In life, as in a play, it is not about how long it lasts, but how well it is played. (Seneca)

Overview

He saw the signs of his death—within himself, on himself, and around him. And with a sign, he went expectantly into dying. C. G. Jung is today considered one of the most important psychotherapists of the early days of scientific psychotherapy. He continued Freud's theories and opened up new areas of the human psyche. Thus, he developed the concept of "archetypes", the "collective unconscious", the complex theory, and founded his own psychological typology. He saw his death as a transition.

C. G. Jung is another great psychotherapist of the first generation who founded his own depth psychology therapy school. In addition to Freud's psychoanalysis and Adler's individual psychology, the "analytical psychology" is considered the third major direction of depth psychological schools. It goes back to the Swiss psychiatrist Carl Gustav Jung.

The story of C. G. Jung initially proceeds quite straightforwardly. He was born on July 26, 1875, in Kesswil on Lake Constance in the Swiss canton of Thurgau into a pastor's family.

His father, Johann Paul Achilles Jung, is a Protestant-Reformed pastor. Originally, the paternal branch of the family comes from the German city of Mainz. For the most part, the Jungs were doctors over several generations, but there were also theologians among them. Carl Gustav's grandfather (who also had the first name Carl Gustav) was so actively involved in the expansion of the University of Basel that a painting of him hung in the old auditorium of the university for a long time.

Carl Gustav's mother Emilie comes from the venerable Swiss family Preiswerk, which also had several—partly quite renowned—theologians. Emilie's father, for example, was a professor of theology, under whom her husband had also studied.

Thus, medicine and religion, natural science and faith have always played a significant role in the families of origin of C. G. Jung.

Just half a year after the birth of little Carl Gustav, the pastor's family moves to Laufen, in the immediate vicinity of the Schaffhausen Rhine Falls. Jung later describes what he remembers from his very early experiences: "My memories begin around the second or third year. I remember the parsonage, the garden, the Buchihüsli, the church, the castle, the Rhine Falls …"

What is important to him are the (re-)memories, i.e., what touches him inwardly. He calls it "the imperishable world that breaks into the perishable one".

From a very early age, C. G. Jung shows a strong tendency towards introversion and dreaming. At the age of 65, he tells in his autobiography about dreams he had as a 3- or 4-year-old.

In 1879, when Carl Gustav is just 4 years old, the pastor's family moves to Kleinhüningen near Basel, because the father is called to the local church community. There the boy also goes to school and practices a kind of double life: On the outside, he manages a more or less normal student life with his classmates. Inside, however, lives "the other", who has a "fatal resistance to life in this world", as he later writes in his autobiography, and who "knew a secret, personal and at the same time superpersonal secret".

He believes that he is "actually in reality two persons". These two sides and the basic attitude later also lead to everything esoteric-occult exerting a great fascination on him. Because already in his childhood, Jung has a strong affinity for symbols, dreams, and mystical or unexplainable experiences.

11.1 Personality No. 1 and No. 2

Thus, in Jung's psyche, "Personality No. 1" and "Personality No. 2" stand opposed as antipodes. This does not have to be a split in the pathological sense, but in analytical psychology, No. 2 is then also later understood as the inner side of the person, in which religion also plays a central role, while

No. 1 is the side that one shows to the outside world and with which one acts in it.

Jung often feels lonely already in childhood, which leads to depressive states repeatedly later in life. During puberty, he probably suffers from a longer, pronounced depression.

11.2 Mother

He feels most understood by his mother, who—despite sometimes suffering from depression herself—radiates an "animal warmth" for him. However, she is also a "dark, large figure, the untouchable authority" for him, who is experienced strangely and mysteriously by the boy at night – also because she feels visited by ghosts on some nights. When she has to undergo treatment in a clinic for a longer period of time, Carl Gustav is accommodated with an unmarried sister of the mother. As a result, Jung is said to have later associated women with unreliability.

11.3 Father

The father is experienced as dutiful, depressive, and introverted. He is also an authority for him, but Carl Gustav always views him with a certain skepticism and finds it difficult to connect with him. Above all, the father's theological duty leads him to the conviction that he does not know what he is preaching. In his opinion, the father – like many theologians – has not had any real religious experiences. Thus, he rejects the church dogmas as well as the school regulations.

11.4 Family

When he is 9 years old, his sister Johanna Gertrud ("Trudi") is born. She will become his long-term secretary later in life.

And there is another family secret: In the Jung family, it is not talked about that there was a son (Paulus) in the family who was born in 1873 (thus 2 years before the birth of Carl Gustav) but only survived a few days. Thus, Carl Gustav is not really the firstborn, but becomes the eldest only due to the early death of his brother.

11.5 Faints

Carl Gustav is 12 years old when he gets into a fight with another boy just before changing to high school and briefly loses consciousness during the brawl. During this faint, a thought suddenly comes to him: "now you don't have to go to school anymore". From this incident, he faints sporadically on the way to school and when trying to do homework. There is a suspicion of epilepsy and C. G. does not have to go to school for 6 months. When one day he hears his father talking to someone about how his son could best support him, he immediately starts helping his father, as Carl Gustav is aware of his family's financial difficulties. After that, he only faints 3 more times and soon the habit of collapsing is completely broken. During this time, he also develops—more or less consciously—rituals, ceremonial actions, and totems that apparently help him cope with difficult situations. Later he writes: "A young man who does not fight and win has missed the best of his youth, and an old man who does not understand the mystery of streams rushing from peaks to valleys is pointless, a spiritual mummy, which is nothing but frozen past."

11.6 High School

From 1886, Carl Gustav attends high school in Basel. Since his schoolmates mostly come from well-to-do families and are generously equipped with pocket money, Jung feels that he is the son of a poor country pastor, who sometimes has to sit in class with holes in his shoe soles and wet socks. This realization leads to a better understanding of his father—and also to pity for him.

From the age of 16, his depressive states improve—probably also because he gets to know the great world of the spirit and important figures of philosophy. He deals with ancient Greek thinkers like Socrates, Plato, Pythagoras, Heraclitus, and later also with other philosophers like Schopenhauer.

11.7 Studies

Jung is not sure whether he should study humanities or natural sciences, as he is interested and fascinated by both.

Apart from purely practical considerations, his namesake grandfather, known for his liberal individualism, is said to have been decisive for his choice to study medicine—and thus a good role model for him.

From 1895, Jung studies medicine in Basel, becomes a member of a fraternity and the "Swiss Zofingia Association", deals with Spiritism, ghost appearances, and attends séances.

When his father dies in 1896, as a young student he has to—at least partially—provide for the maintenance of his mother and sister. He completes his medical state examination at the turn of the century in 1900.

11.8 Burghölzli

In the same year, he moves to Zurich and becomes an assistant to the famous psychiatrist Eugen Bleuler, who works at the "Burghölzli", the psychiatric clinic of the University of Zurich.

The Burghölzli is a great place for his professional development in the field of psychiatry, as it is known at the time as one of the leading psychiatric clinics in all of Europe. The hospital is located in a large and well-equipped building on the Holzhügel (hence the name Burghölzli) in the southeast of Zurich. Since 1842, it has been operating as a care facility for chronic, old, and incurable mentally ill patients. The psychiatric reformer Auguste-Henri Forel took over the management of the Burghölzli in 1879 and was director there for almost 20 years. Under him, it was recognized throughout Europe for its psychiatric treatments and research.

Over time, this care facility is transformed into a—for its time—modern psychiatric clinic, with a close connection to the university and above all with a humane treatment of mentally ill patients. Eugen Bleuler, who takes over the Burghölzli after Forel in 1898, continues his work. The Bleuler era, which lasts until 1927, is widely regarded as the most revolutionary time of the hospital, especially because of the successful application of psychoanalytic theories and the groundbreaking work of C. G. Jung.

11.9 Dissertation

At the Burghölzli, Jung deals with the phenomenon of split personality and completes his dissertation in 1902. Topic: *On the Psychology and Pathology of So-Called Occult Phenomena*. In 1905, he becomes the permanent senior physician of the hospital, qualifies as a university lecturer and for several years gives lectures on psychoneuroses and psychology, which are very well attended.

11.10 Starting a Family

C. G. Jung marries Emma Rauschenbach in February 1903, who comes from a wealthy Schaffhausen family. The fortune Emma brings into the marriage is an important prerequisite for the free development of C. G. Jung's creativity and his research work.

Emma is strongly interested in natural sciences, but is also fascinated by the Grail legend. She is an important conversation partner and competent critic for Jung, whose manuscripts she partly edits and writes. From 1930, she also works as an analyst herself. The couple have a total of four daughters and one son.

11.11 Jung's Relationship with Freud

Probably at the suggestion of Bleuler, Jung reads Freud's *Interpretation of Dreams* as early as 1900 and is initially not particularly impressed. Only when he describes the case of an obsessive-compulsive disorder in his habilitation thesis, which he investigates with association experiments and successfully treats with Freud's psychoanalytic method, does he note in his habilitation that his association experiment could be helpful for Freud's psychoanalysis.

In April 1906, he sends his diagnostic association studies to Freud. This marks the beginning of a 7-year, regular and very intense correspondence between the two.

When he visits Freud in Vienna on March 3, 1907, the two men engage in deep professional discussions for 13 hours and are highly impressed with each other. A long-lasting, close friendship develops.

Jung is considered the "crown prince of psychoanalysis" until 1912. Since Freud, who is almost 20 years older than Jung, thinks highly of his "adoptive son" and protects him on many levels, he undertakes a several-week trip to the USA with him in 1909, where they participate in a conference at Clark University.

Finally, in 1910, Jung becomes the first president of the "International Psychoanalytical Association". Originally, Freud probably intended to have him elected as president for life—against which, however, there were strong protests from the Viennese colleagues, which led to Jung being elected for a 2-year term.

Freud also appreciates that Jung, as a "Christian and pastor's son", joins his theory—not least because this changes the image of psychoanalysis—that it is primarily a Jewish affair.

11.12 Points of Contention

However, at the turn of the year 1912/1913, there is a break between the two men.

The tensions between Jung and Freud become apparent when Jung publishes his text *Transformations and Symbols of the Libido*. Various significant disagreements emerge, especially when it comes to the assessment of the libido. Jung agrees with Freud that the libido is an important source of personal growth, but unlike Freud, he does not see it as solely responsible for the formation of a person's core personality. Jung believes that a person's personal development is also influenced by factors that have nothing to do with sexuality. Instead, he emphasizes the "collective unconscious"—memories and ideas inherited from ancestors and expressed in the various myths of cultures.

Further points of contention between the two are their differing views on the unconscious: According to Jung, Freud's concept of the unconscious is incomplete, inflexible, and unnecessarily negative. Freud sees the unconscious only as a reservoir of suppressed emotions and desires. Jung, on the other hand, believes that there is both a personal unconscious and a collective unconscious. And a "psychoid"—a kind of overarching form of the unconscious, a soul-like layer—which is close to the realm of drives.

Freud can no longer accept Jung's divergent views. But Jung sticks to his differing views on Freud's theory, which Freud no longer wants to tolerate. And so it comes to separation and demarcation. Freud declares "that he could not regard the works and explanations of the Swiss as a legitimate continuation of psychoanalysis". Jung responds with sharp—also personal—accusations, whereupon Freud formally ends their friendship in writing in January 1913. The last personal encounter between Jung and Freud probably took place in September 1913, when both attended the 4th International Psychoanalytic Congress in Munich, but no longer spoke to each other. This is not easy for Freud, but the separation from Freud is also not easy for Jung. He undergoes a painful psychological transformation, which is exacerbated by the outbreak of World War I. Jung later says about this: "Freud had a neurosis."

11.13 Analytical Psychology

Jung now calls his school "analytical psychology" and publishes numerous books in the following years. He increasingly distances himself from Freud's psychoanalysis. Sexuality and aggression play only a minor role in analytical psychology. He incorporates philosophical questions, mystical and religious experiences into his method and is far less deterministic.

In addition to the personal unconscious, Jung assumes something that all people share—the collective unconscious, in which universal symbols and myths are found, which Jung refers to as "archetypes".

The goal of Jung's treatment method is "individuation", the maturation and differentiation of one's own person. However, this is not as easy as one might think: "There are far more people who are afraid of the unconscious than one would expect. They are even afraid of their own shadow." (Jung 2011, p. 42).

11.14 The Scandalous Affair: Sabina Spielrein

Even during the correspondence in the years 1906 and 1907, Jung discusses with Freud the relationship to the Russian-born Sabina Spielrein. She was a patient of C. G. Jung at Burghölzli from 1904-1907 with the diagnosis: hysteria. During the therapy, a strong transference and countertransference situation develops. Jung first mentions the patient in the correspondence with Freud in 1906 because she "wants a child from him". This brings the topic of transference and countertransference in psychoanalysis to the fore. Some analysts suspect that this may have been the reason for Freud to insist that anyone who wanted to practice as a psychoanalyst must have undergone a "training analysis" beforehand.

From 1908 onwards—at least according to diary entries and letters—an intimate relationship develops between Jung and Spielrein.

Spielrein later becomes a psychoanalyst herself and is the first woman to earn a doctorate on a distinctly psychoanalytic topic. Because of the affair with Jung, she had direct written contact with Sigmund Freud and goes to Vienna for some time, later participates in the legendary "Wednesday Societies" and becomes a member of the Vienna Psychoanalytic Association.

This relationship is revisited and scandalized in the feature film "A Dangerous Method" by David Cronenberg in 2015 (over 100 years later), full of speculation and sensationalism.

11.15 Toni Wolff

Another woman plays an important role in Jung's life: Antonia Wolff (called "Toni") starts working for Jung in 1912, becomes his closest confidante from 1913 onwards and later his lover. Some refer to Wolff as "Jung's analyst", who was especially his main support during the time of separation from Freud. Others call her "Jung's second wife", as the relationship with her is intimate on many levels. The marriage with Emma continues and often Toni, Emma, and Carl Gustav appear together. As if there were no conflicts.

11.16 Private Practice and Travels

In the period after his separation from Freud, Jung establishes his private practice in Küsnacht, further elaborates what is to be understood by analytical psychology (also in distinction to psychoanalysis), writes several books in the following years, and travels extensively. He visits the Pueblo tribes in America, travels to North and East Africa and to India. Also in Switzerland, he deals with various topics: the unconscious, with dreams and fantasies, but also with Taoism, with alchemy and various esoteric practices.

11.17 The Reputation Rises

In doing so, Jung becomes increasingly well-known in professional circles. His reputation overall increases. Thus, in 1929 he is invited by the "International General Medical Society for Psychotherapy" (IAÄGP) to give one of the main lectures at the annual congress. In 1930 he becomes the 2nd chairman of the association, in 1933 chairman and editor of the *Zentralblatt für Psychotherapie*.

11.18 National Socialism

However, this also brings him under suspicion of currying favor with the National Socialists, who had by then seized power in Germany. Thus, the Nazis repeatedly demand declarations of loyalty from Jung. In the early 1930s, there are various statements from him sympathizing with the "Germanic spirit" and "Jewish psychology," which he later wants to be understood as "value-neutral." Privately, after the 2nd World War, Jung apologized to his Jewish colleagues and friends for his earlier statements.

His later distance from the Nazi ideology is also evident in the fact that Jung's works were put on the black list in the German Reich from 1939 onwards.

11.19 Honesty and Humility

Carl Gustav Jung is considered by his employees and patients to be an open, honest, and humble person. Marie Louise von Franz, who was not only a direct student of C. G. Jung for a long time, but also a close collaborator since the mid-1930s, tells me in an interview:

> **Interview**
>
> "I knew him the last 28 years of his life, he died in '61. And I would say—I was 18 years old when I first met him. My first impression was, of course, 'this is a Methuselah'. He was only 58 at the time, but for an 18-year-old that's a Methuselah. I was deeply impressed. I had the feeling that this is the most honest person I have ever met. With this person I could talk about everything, without him cowardly evading, as teachers and most adults usually do."

Marie Louise von Franz studied classical philology, translated texts from Greek and Latin for him. She attests to Jung: "A great humility. An almost too great humility. He sometimes accused me of being too humble, and later he said:

> **Interview**
>
> 'I often have to pat myself on the shoulder and say, you are no longer the pastor's boy from Kesswil, you are now Jung.' … I would say, the essence is—and this is already in this first impression of honesty—his work is what he lived. And he lived every word of what he said. There is this discrepancy, which bothers one so much with Nietzsche or Kierkegaard, it was not present with him. He always drew the consequence that what he said, he also applied to himself and lived. … His goal was also to live as consciously as possible. So he means: 'An **inner** situation that one has not made **conscious** appears outside as fate.'"

11.20 Near-Death Experiences

In February 1944, the nearly 70-year-old Jung slips on an extended, solitary hike and falls awkwardly—many kilometers away from his apartment. He suffers a fracture of the fibula and drags himself with the last of his strength on icy ground to the nearest house and is taken from there to a private clinic. He has to lie still, which initially makes him quite happy. After about 10 days, he suffers a severe heart embolism and two more lung embolisms. He falls into a deep unconsciousness and finds himself for a few days on the threshold of death. He has visions and deliriums of unprecedented grandeur. He thinks he is floating high in space and sees the planet Earth far below him. Temples appear and a priest-doctor tells him that he must not yet leave the Earth, as he still has a message to deliver. Jung is disappointed.

The work he is writing at this time, *Mysterium Coiunctionis*, is strongly influenced by this experience. Marie Louise von Franz, who worked on the text:

> **Interview**
>
> "He later told me, when we saw each other again and sat at the manuscript, he said: 'What I have written is correct. I don't need to change anything about it, but now I know how real it is.' As if he had now experienced the reality of it …
>
> Through these death visions, which he reports in his memories, these visions have confirmed to him that what he wrote really exists—in full reality."

11.21 Suffering Success

It is certainly not only due to Jung's personality that analytical psychology is becoming increasingly well-known. After his many studies and the multitude of publications on *Psychological Types, Symbols of Transformation, The Archetypes, Psychology and Religion* and *The Dynamics of the Unconscious*, the analytical psychology is gaining more and more recognition worldwide.

The C. G. Jung Institute in Zurich was founded in 1948. However, Carl Gustav slowly withdraws, as he "suffers success". Marie Louise von Franz recalls:

> **Interview**
>
> "Yes, his vitality slowly faded. He became tired more quickly. He was often sick. He frequently had the flu and then disappeared into bed. ... And then he was often tired, and he repeatedly complained to me, 'I am an old ruin, I am an old car that is leaking oil'. Once he said: 'I have never been old in my life. That is terribly difficult to learn.' And then he consciously began to withdraw from his enormous workload ...
>
> And his main conflict was that the work was chasing him, and he was, so to speak, constantly fighting a defensive battle against too many patients, too many letters, too many demands. He had to endure a kind of rearguard action ...
>
> And he was always happy when he could sit in the sun in his beloved Bollingen and then cook for himself and the world left him in peace ...
>
> So I would say, he had not lost his interest in the world, but he tried to reduce his engagement in the world. He tried to detach himself and stay out of it, which was very difficult for him because of his good heart and his temperament."

Jung preferred to be in Bollingen. This was the place on the upper Lake Zurich where he had built a tower with his own hands in 1923. There was no electricity and no running water, but Jung liked to retreat there when he wanted to be completely alone or wanted to write.

11.22 Death of the Wife

When his wife Emma dies in 1955, for Jung the time of farewell, of the end of life, begins. His student and private secretary Aniela Jaffe describes him at this time as fragile and slightly stooped, but still full of a "radiating power".

Only smaller works are created. However, he continues to answer letters and give interviews. He also works manually in and on his tower in Bollingen. He feels that his scientific work is essentially done.

Marie Louise von Franz describes:

> **Interview**
>
> "He had the feeling that the harvest is fully brought in. And what he suffered was the correspondence in the last months. It became more and more burdensome for him. ... He had a minor stroke shortly before the end and therefore could not speak well for a few days, and then he triumphantly took the mail and threw it into the wastebasket and indicated in a gesture: 'Now I don't need to do this anymore.' So he was also glad to finally be able to lay down the burden."

11.23 Preparations for Dying

In the last years of his life, Jung dealt with death and dying. And in the circle of students who surrounded him especially in the last years, he spoke about it several times. Marie Louise von Franz recalls:

> **Interview**
>
> "He said: 'I am prepared for death', and in the sense of looking forward joyfully—as he himself writes—looking forward joyfully to the new adventure. So an enormous scientific curiosity about what is coming, so a real adventurer's curiosity. ... I would not say 'longing for death', but a certain joyful expectation: 'Now something very interesting is coming, now something exciting is coming, now I will experience great things that I do not yet know.' And on the other hand, pain of parting. So simply both, the opposites."

11.24 Initial Dreams

Jung has always, and not just before his death, strongly believed in the messages from dreams. Significant dreams that want to tell him something about the future, he calls "initial dreams". Frau von Franz recalls:

> **Interview**
>
> "He told me, 'I had an important dream: I was in the afterlife. I was heading towards the afterlife Bollingen.' Of course, this was something he didn't need to explain to me, namely, that he had dreams throughout his life that there is a Bollingen in the afterlife, which was for him an image of the self or the divine soul core.
>
> And he was heading towards this Bollingen, and it was all made of gold. And he held a key, a golden key, in his hand and knew he was going there, and a voice said: 'Now everything is ready, now you can move in.' So everything was ready for his arrival, for his death ..."

At another point, he tells Marie Louise von Franz about:

> **Interview**
>
> "A wolverine mother, who showed her wolverine child on a cliff by the sea how to swim, thus teaching swimming. And he did not interpret this dream. I then interpreted it myself. Of course, I immediately more or less understood the dream and therefore became very sad."

In another dream, he sees an "Ouroboros", a snake biting its own tail, thus forming a circle. Some call it the "snake of eternity"—a symbol for the eternal cycle, infinity.

11.25 Death Wedding Procession

When he realized that his last days had come, he had his student Barbara Hannah drive him through the streets of his hometown Küsnacht one last time to say goodbye. During this, his vehicle crosses the same wedding procession 3 times. His student concludes from this that this was his "death wedding procession"—the mythical representation of the union of life and death.

Barbara Hannah had a sad feeling at this noticeably frequent encounter of weddings, because it could also be a death omen. For in many myths, fairy tales and folk songs, death is often portrayed as a mystical wedding, as a union of opposites. In analytical psychology, it is a union with the inner feminine ("anima") in a man, and in a woman the union with the inner masculine ("animus"), thus a becoming whole, a completion.

11.26 Saying Goodbye

Three weeks before his death, Jung suffers another minor stroke, which makes speaking difficult for him. But he still receives all those who are important to him and says goodbye. Marie Louise von Franz describes:

> **Interview**
>
> "He had most of the people who were important to him come one more time and said goodbye to them. But he didn't say it directly. He said goodbye to me ..., but we didn't speak it out. We talked about this and that, but it was perfectly clear that he knew this was our farewell visit. And I also knew it was the last time I would see him alive.
>
> I had the feeling he wanted to have contact one more time to say certain things, important things. So in that sense, he prepared his detachment from this world ...
>
> Or, for example, he said goodbye to his son. One afternoon, as his son sat by his sickbed, he said: 'Get the best bottle of wine.' It was sunset, and then he said: 'Pour me a glass and you a glass', and then they toasted to the sunset. But again he didn't say anything. It was like a ritual, but it was clear."

11.27 "How wonderful …"

There follows another minor stroke and Jung has to stay in bed for the last week. When he occasionally woke up, he seemed a little disappointed that he was still there and consciousness was returning. His employee von Franz:

> **Interview**
>
> "'He hoped to have already gone.' In moments of mental absence, he muttered a few times: 'how wonderful, how wonderful …'"

Marie Louise von Franz, who was not present at Jung's hour of death, says that those present report that Jung lay very quietly in the last minutes, took a deep sigh with some effort, closed his eyes himself and extinguished without a death struggle.

11.28 Hour of Death

Carl Gustav Jung dies on June 6, 1961 around 3:45 pm—7 weeks before his 86th birthday. Shortly after his death, a violent storm brews over Lake Zurich. A lightning bolt strikes a poplar on the shore of his garden and splits it. An unusual phenomenon, as normally the water attracts the lightning and it does not strike the trees on the shore. Some of his students see this as a symbol. For Jungians can interpret this and other peculiarities that happened at Jung's hour of death in the sense of "synchronicity".

11.29 Synchronicity and Reincarnation

Synchronicity is also a term that Jung developed, and it means that special things happen simultaneously without a causal connection, thereby creating a symbolic connection that is meaningful.

But C. G. Jung actually had little time for pathos. He wanted to stay in death after death and see what happens there. He left life to the living. Marie Louise von Franz says:

> **Interview**
>
> "Reincarnation is possible for Jung. He has seen traces of it in certain dreams. But he is not sure. Jung was a passionate scientist until the end. He wanted to observe and see where it goes. And he had open questions. He was quite convinced that individual life continues, but he was not 100% sure."

He rather agreed with the Jewish proverb: "You are closer to God when you ask a question than when you give an answer."

11.30 Funeral

So the operation at the C. G. Jung Institute continued as normal. Only for the funeral was it closed for a day. Jung had said much earlier to Marie Louise von Franz:

> **Interview**
>
> "I am introverted. Such external ceremonies mean nothing to me. I have sat through them and shielded myself internally and was glad when they were over. I am not interested in funerals. … Kings are buried in gold and silver—I will be buried under mountains of paper, under endless biographies and obituaries."

On June 9, 1961, Carl Gustav Jung is buried in the cemetery in Küsnacht.

And Marie Louise von Franz had the fantasy during Jung's funeral that if Jung were there now, he would nudge her with his elbow and say: "Look, look, how ridiculous and crazy they all are and now they all make their speeches!"

For his tombstone, he had chosen the same saying that was also engraved above the threshold of his house:

"Vocatus atque non vocatus deus aderit." "Called or not called, God will be there."

11.31 Conclusion

Carl Gustav Jung, the visionary, the "mystic", the supernatural, deals most clearly with death and especially with his own death. Basically, he prepares for his death for 17 years of his life—since his heart attack. His thesis of the collective unconscious turns into a wonder at the moment of agony that he is still conscious. Jung faces death prepared, curious about a new adventure, for him death is not the end. He considers reincarnation possible. Does the human being dissolve in his "shadow" at the moment of his death?

Bibliography

Franz, Marie Louise von: Traum und Tod, München 1934 (Kösel)
Franz, Marie Louise von, Frey-Rohn, L., Jaffe, A.: Im Umkreis des Todes, Zürich 1980 (Daimon)
Freud, Sigmund, Jung, Carl Gustav: Briefwechsel, Frankfurt 1984 (Fischer TB)
Hannah, Barbara: C. G. Jung – Sein Leben und Wirken, Fellbach 1982 (Bonz)
Jaffe Aniela: Aus C. G. Jungs letzten Jahren, in: Aufsätze zur Psychologie, Zürich 1982 (Daimon)
Jung, Carl Gustav: Der Mensch und seine Symbole, Olten 1979 (Walter)
Jung, Carl Gustav: Bewußtes und Unbewußtes, Frankfurt 1972 (Fischer TB)
Jung, Carl Gustav: Die Dynamik des Unbewußten, Ostfildern 2011 (Patmos)
Wehr, Gerhard: C. G. Jung, Reinbek 1969 (rororo – Monographien)
Wehr, Gerhard: Carl Gustav Jung – Leben, Werk, München 1985 (Kösel)
Interview mit Dr. Marie Louise von Franz, direkte Schülerin von C. G. Jung (1985)

12

Interlude VI: Finiteness—Lifetime—Dying Time (Small Exercises)

Contents

12.1 The Temporal Questions 126
12.2 How Do I Want to Die? 126
12.3 And After? 127
Further Reading 127

> This article is about a few small exercises that have to do with one's own finiteness and how to appropriately use the remaining lifetime (however long it may be).

I have nothing against death. I just don't want to be there when it happens. (Woody Allen)

Someone once said: "Life is like drawing without an eraser." What's on the sheet (of life) is on it. What has happened, has happened. You can't change the past. But you can draw lessons from it for the remaining time and try to change what can still be changed.

Because when you look at life from the end, you can ask yourself:

What is actually a good, a successful life for me?

I'll gladly tell you my opinion on this: For me personally, a successful life is a meaningful and purposeful life. Sensual means that I (short-term) enjoy my life. Purposeful means that I see a (long-term) purpose in my life—whether I do this with the help of an adopted religion, a philosophy, or a self-made system of meaning.

12.1 The Temporal Questions

When this topic comes up with a patient in psychotherapy (which is not so rare), I sometimes give them a few questions for the next sessions:

- What would you do if you only had **one hour** left to live?
- What would you do if you only had **one day** left to live?
- What would you do if you only had **one month** left to live?
- What would you do if you only had **one year** left to live?
- What would you do if you had **5 years** left to live?
- What would you do if you had **20 years** left to live?

Sometimes I give the patient only one question per session, sometimes several or even all. It depends on how much time someone wants and can take to deal with their own finiteness and death.

Basically, it's about the question: Do I give myself, my life, and my lifetime another chance for change—or am I at the mercy of the basic pattern, the rut, the "autopilot" that governs me? What do I want (and can) still do? What do I definitely want to experience?

12.2 How Do I Want to Die?

Even if our way of dying is not really planable, we are allowed to have wishes about how we would like to die. Specifically: How do I actually wish to die?

- Gently and slowly drift off to sleep? ("Wake up and be dead?")
- Quickly and without a death struggle? ("Heart attack: ruck zuck")
- Pain-free?
- As a result of a fulfilled life? ("What is a fulfilled life for me?")
- When I have everything sorted out? ("leave a well-ordered field behind")
- In the arms of my lover?
- Alone and thrown back on myself?
- One with me and my life story?
- Knowing and wise?
- Not wake up after an orgasm (the "little death")?

- As a result of a death struggle?
- Just dissolve myself? Fade away? Leave? Fade?
- Or how?

Remembering this: Not all wishes are fulfilled …

12.3 And After?

- What should remain of me?
- How should others remember me?
- Who do I definitely not want to be forgotten by?
- What should be laughed about at the wake?
- What should the eulogist say about me?
- What should be written about me in the obituary?
- What should be written on my gravestone?
- What do I want to leave behind?
- What else is important?

Note: If you are at peace with yourself, it is easier to accept that you do not know what is coming.

Further Reading

Keleman, Stanley: Lebe dein Sterben, Hamburg 1977 (Isko-Press)
Korp, Harald-Alexander: Am Ende ist nicht Schluss mit lustig, Gütersloh 2014 (Gütersloher Verlagshaus)
Mulford, Prentice: Unfug des Lebens und des Sterbens, Frankfurt 1977 (Fischer TB)
Schultz, Hans Jürgen (Hrsg.): Letzte Tage, Stuttgart 1983 (Kreuz)
Watts, Alan: Tod, Basel 1977 (Sphinx)

13

Karlfried Graf Dürckheim (1896–1988): Endured Pain During Conscious Transition

Contents

13.1	First Experience with Death	131
13.2	Military Service in the 1st World War	131
13.3	Studies	132
13.4	Religion and Mysticism	132
13.5	University of Leipzig	132
13.6	Nazi Era	133
13.7	Japan and Zen	133
13.8	Todtmoos-Rütte	134
13.9	Initiatic Therapy	134
13.10	Rütte Impulse	136
13.11	Appreciation	136
13.12	Limitations	137
13.13	The Door Opens Inward	137
13.14	Daily Routine	138
13.15	In the Face of Death	138
13.16	Hour of Death	139
13.17	Conclusion	139
Further Reading		140

© The Author(s), under exclusive license to Springer-Verlag GmbH, DE, part of Springer Nature 2024
W. Gross, *As One Lives, So One Dies*, https://doi.org/10.1007/978-3-662-70061-7_13

> **Trailer**
>
> Up to this point we have reported on how great psychotherapists have lived and how they have died. We have also explained how outsiders have talked about how the therapists in question have faced their death.
>
> This chapter is to report on a man who told me about how he is facing his death and preparing for it before he died.
>
> It is Karlfried Graf Dürckheim, who together with Maria Hippius developed a psychotherapy method in the small Black Forest village of Todtmoos-Rütte, which is called "initiatic therapy".
>
> Before he arrives there, he goes through many years of wandering and transformation—offspring of nobility, front officer, psychology professor, NS diplomat, "never again a soldier", psychotherapist, mystic, Zen master, meditation teacher and soul guide.

God sleeps in the stones, he breathes in the plants, he dreams in the animals and he awakens in humans. (Rumi)

> Some people hear the sound of their inner voice very early on. Even if they deal with very different topics on the outer level and move and prove themselves in very different life worlds, this inner melody does not leave them. This deep experience of a transcendent reality is the mysticism in the person presented in this chapter of the book. From an early age, the person in question has enlightenment experiences and embarks—despite many detours and wrong turns—on the search for an intensification of this other state of being.

Karlfried Graf Dürckheim (his full name: Karl Friedrich Alfred Heinrich Ferdinand Maria Graf Eckbrecht von Dürckheim-Montmartin) is born on October 24, 1896 as a member of a noble family in Munich. His father—Friedrich Georg Michael Maria Graf Eckbrecht von Dürckheim-Montmartin—and his mother Sophie Evalina Ottilie Charlotte von Kusserow belong to the old nobility circles of Bavaria.

Ancestors of the paternal noble family can be traced back to the 12th century, i.e. back to the time of Emperor Frederick I ("Barbarossa").

In the maternal line, his origin goes back to the 15th century to the Jewish Rothschild family.

Karlfried thus has a long and significant family tree to show: For example, Karlfried's maternal grandfather was the Prussian diplomat and politician Heinrich von Kusserow, whose mother was a daughter of the Jewish banker Salomon Oppenheim and who himself married Antonie Springer, a daughter of the also Jewish banker and merchant Ernst Springer.

13.1 First Experience with Death

Karlfried grows up on the family estate in Steingaden and has a very early first encounter with death. In a conversation I had with him in 1986, he tells me:

> **Interview**
>
> "One can say that my life began with a strange encounter with death. As a one-and-a-half-year-old child, I was carried into my grandmother's death room on the arm of my nanny and she let my head touch the head of the dead. So my life began with the encounter with death. I still feel that today. … It is a clear memory, a very simple feeling. It smelled of wax, the candles were burning. And I can't say that I experienced a great shock. I was only 1.5 years old. It is only the external fact to state that my life began with a physical touch of death."

Karlfried Graf Dürckheim attends the grammar school in Koblenz and Weimar, graduates—as not uncommon in wartime—with an emergency high school diploma in 1914. He participates in the 1st World War as an 18-year-old in the body regiment of the Bavarian army.

13.2 Military Service in the 1st World War

Since Graf Dürckheim is still integrated into the collective structures of his family of origin at this time, military service in the 1st World War is not a question: It is service to the fatherland for him.

Dürckheim experiences the battles at Verdun without being wounded and is a lieutenant at the end of the World War. In our interview, he also reports on this:

> **Interview**
>
> "At 18 years old I was in the war and was at the front for 4 years. I am one of two who came out of this hell unwounded and have experienced many situations in which the death was accepted by me …
>
> Imagine a drumfire that you have to go through. Something like that was called a 'curtain of grenades' at the time. And I shouted to my men: Jump into the hole that has just been formed by a grenade. It is unlikely that another grenade will fall into the same hole in the next moment …
>
> This terrible war … Fort Douaumont for example, that was one of the positions conquered by our regiment. These are unforgettable experiences—through the death of so many people, who I saw fall right next to me …
>
> I had a personal assignment and had to go to the very front every day, where our people were lying. The terrain there was simply churned up by corpses. Everywhere a leg or an arm stuck out of the ground. So it was really a constant encounter with death."

13.3 Studies

After the 1st World War, Dürckheim fought in a Freikorps against the Munich Soviet Republic in 1919. He first studied National Economics, and from 1919–1923 Philosophy and Psychology, initially in Munich.

During this time, he moved in a circle of intellectuals and artists and associated with, among others, Rainer Maria Rilke and Ludwig Klages.

13.4 Religion and Mysticism

At the beginning of the 1920s he was intensively involved with religious studies and the psychology of religion. He began with mystical exercises and studied the texts of Meister Eckhardt and other—also Far Eastern—mystics.

According to his own statements, while reading the Tao-Te-King, the most important scripture of Taoism, he experienced a kind of enlightenment ("satori").

He had a deep friendship with the philosopher Ferdinand Weinhandl and his wife, the writer Margarete Weinhandl. He moved with the Weinhandls to Kiel and lived there in a shared apartment.

In 1923, he received his doctorate from the University of Kiel with a thesis on *Forms of Experience—Approaches to an Analytical Situation Psychology* and graduated with a Dr. phil.

In the same year, he married Enja von Hattingberg and went with her to Italy for a year in 1924. There he studied art and continued to be financed by his parents.

13.5 University of Leipzig

From 1925 onwards, he worked at the Psychological Institute of the University of Leipzig.

From 1927, he was an assistant to the founder of the 2nd Leipzig School, the holistic psychologist Felix Krüger.

In his studies and teaching, Dürckheim primarily devoted himself to "thought psychology" and the qualitative "forms of experience" of the psyche. In Felix Krueger, the successor to the founding father of scientific psychology, Wilhelm Wundt in Leipzig, he found support and recognition for his approach. Dürckheim's concept of "unity philosophy" can be fruitfully combined with Krueger's holistic psychology.

On February 17, 1930, he qualified as a professor in Leipzig with the topic *Experience Reality and its Understanding*. From 1930-1932, he taught psychology at the Bauhaus in Dessau. At the same time, in 1931, he took up a professorship at the Pedagogical Academy in Breslau and moved to the University of Kiel in 1932. During this time of the world economic crisis, his parents lost the family estate in Steingaden.

13.6 Nazi Era

In November 1933, Dürckheim (more or less voluntarily) signed the confession of the German university professors to Adolf Hitler.

In 1934, Dürkheim was sent by Reich Education Minister Rust to explore the German diaspora in South Africa.

Through personal connections, Dürckheim moved to the office of Foreign Minister Ribbentrop in 1935. He was even introduced to Hitler and later arranged a meeting between Hitler and Lord Beaverbrook.

However, due to the racial laws, he lost the permission to continue teaching in the civil service. According to the Nuremberg Laws, Dürkheim was considered a "quarter Jew", which is why he was dismissed by Ribbentrop in December 1937.

13.7 Japan and Zen

Nevertheless, he remains in public service. With the explicitly defined task of "caring for Germans abroad," he is sent to Japan for the first time in 1938 as an employee of the Foreign Office's press department. From 1940–1945, he works in Japan with interruptions and encounters Zen Buddhism and its practices there. Since this time, he has been meditating and practicing archery. During this time, Dürkheim has another enlightenment experience ("satori") during a tea ceremony.

In parallel, he delves further into the Christian mysticism of Meister Eckhart.

In 1940, his wife dies in Germany. He briefly returns to Germany for the funeral and to report. He returns to Japan with the explicit mission to maintain contact with Japanese scientists and contribute to the research of the "foundations of Japanese education". During this time, he also likely propagates for the National Socialism. For example, on Hitler's birthday, he gives a 2-hour speech on the topic at the German-Japanese Cultural Institute in Kumamoto.

In 1944, Dürckheim is awarded the War Merit Cross 2nd Class.

"The immeasurable suffering that is in Germany today will elevate the German people one step higher and bring them even closer to themselves, and give birth to deeper life attitudes," he writes to a friend in the last days of the war. The war becomes a personal individuation experience for him, from which he partly develops his therapy.

However, during the years in Japan, a profound change takes place in Count Dürckheim's attitude, which has been developing since his early childhood:

Although he has long carried the deep experience of a transcendent reality within him, this becomes more and more apparent. Through meditation, spiritual training, and consciousness work, the goal is to turn away from traditional bonds and conscience formations.

With the collapse of the Third Reich and the end of World War II, he is interned in Japan for 16 months and is released from there without charge.

In 1947, the American occupiers bring him back to Germany. During this time, he goes through a deep depression, which he later retrospectively sees as an important time of preparation for his future life and his life's mission.

13.8 Todtmoos-Rütte

Upon returning to Germany, Dürckheim meets the widowed Maria Hippius again, whom he knows from his time working at the University of Leipzig. She becomes his second life partner and he moves to her in Todtmoos in the Black Forest in 1948.

In 1951, the couple can affordably acquire a house in Rütte, a district of Todtmoos, as "have-nots". This later becomes known as the "Doctor's House" and is the nucleus of the "existential psychological education and meeting place—the School for Initiatic Therapy". Together with Hippius, Dürckheim develops his initiatic therapy into a unique therapy concept.

Don't believe everything you think. (Zen)

13.9 Initiatic Therapy

Initiatic therapy merges various psychological directions:

It is influenced by depth psychology (Dürckheim completed his training analysis with Gustav Richard Heyer)—especially by the analytical psychology of Carl Gustav Jung. Like him, Dürckheim integrates religious, spiritual, and mystical elements into therapy. However, Dürckheim is much more body-oriented in his therapeutic practice than Jung. One of his favorite sentences:

> The body (Körper) is what you have. The body (Leib) is what you are.

With this, he is close to the Reichian body psychotherapy methods, both directions try to influence the mental state of a person by dissolving bodily tensions through body therapeutic methods. But Dürckheim is more careful with the body than the sometimes brutal Reichians. In Rütte, the work is called "personal body therapy".

In addition, parts of his holistic psychological training from his Leipzig time are used. So there are also similarities with and borrowings from the Gestalt therapy of Fritz Perls.

In addition, elements from the psychodrama of J. L. Moreno can be found in initiatic therapy, such as role-playing with its various techniques, "empty chair", "role exchange", "doubling", "catathymic scene" ...

And above all, aspects of the visual arts—the "guided drawing" (developed by his partner Maria Hippius), painting, working in the clay field, calligraphic ink drawing etc. are also incorporated into this form of therapy, as well as music and movement—and last but not least (Zen-) meditation.

All aim at initiation, the mystical experience. Count Dürckheim tells me in an interview:

Interview

"The term 'initiatic therapy' probably only exists here in Rütte. It refers to a therapy based on an initiatic experience. What is an initiatic experience? It is a mystical experience that is not meant to remain a beautiful memory, but rather contains a mission:

Now you have experienced something unusual. This is not meant to be a beautiful memory, but to set out on the path to changing your life. For example, place an initiatic exercise at the center of your life, which you practice again and again, and try to become who you really are, who testifies in this world what you have just experienced of the transcendent. This is how you prove yourself as a person. Because the word person comes from per-sonare = to sound through. The transcendent should therefore sound through you. Such a person is for me the witness of the transcendent in the world ...

In principle, I would say that the willingness to die is actually the gate to the secret, to the intimate. Often it is only through pain that one enters another dimension. And so initiations are exercises that lead through death. They are initiations into a new dimension."

To avoid misunderstanding: Initiatic therapy is not a call to suicide, but a call to change. The Sufis, the mystics of Islam, say: "Die before you die", that is, change for the better.

Gradually, a slowly but steadily growing community of people with different orientations and imprints is developing in Rütte. If in the 1960s it was still rather stormy confrontations with politically oriented 68ers, which even led to the founding of a commune in Rütte, the first employees grew up in the 1970s.

During this time, Count Dürckheim publishes a whole series of books on the topics of meditation, Zen Buddhism, Transcendence.

13.10 Rütte Impulse

In the 1980s, the number of employees rises to over 60. Many of them take the "Rütte impulse" and establish practices, centers, and institutes in other regions—within and outside of Germany—or work in clinics and social institutions.

After 35 years of living together and working together, Count Dürckheim and Maria Hippius marry in 1985.

Two years before Count Dückheim's death, in 1986, he and Maria Hippius leave a legacy to the employees. It is a pyramidal model in which the institution "Existential Psychological Education and Meeting Place—the School for Initiatic Therapy" should be structured through various institutions and committees.

13.11 Appreciation

Gradually, public recognition for the venerable and yet so modern mystic Count Dürckheim sets in—not least for his bridging between Western and Eastern anthropology, philosophy, and psychology and the Eastern wisdoms that he brought to Europe together with his friend, the Jesuit Father Hugo Makibi Enomiya-Lassalle. The sale of his books and the number of publications about him increase. He becomes an honorary citizen of Todtmoos. Television films and radio broadcasts honor him. He receives the Federal Cross of Merit 1st Class and the Humboldt Plaque.

13.12 Limitations

Count Dürckheim has been gradually going blind since 1970. He said in an interview with me in 1986:

> **Interview**
>
> "I can hardly see anything anymore. For example, I can barely recognize you. When I look in your direction, I first see everything black. I see a light burning here, but in order for me to see anything at all, I have to look very closely and then I only see a contour, a figure. I don't know if it's a man or a woman. I might recognize that by the voice …
>
> My hearing is still quite good at the moment, but my walking is getting worse and worse. I have just spent 14 days in a clinic to fix a disturbance in my right leg, to some extent at least. But walking is getting worse and worse. That's hard for me. And so I can notice daily or weekly how I am decreasing—in physical strength.
>
> I have trouble going uphill, here into my little house on top of the hill. And downhill is even worse, because I feel it in my knee.
>
> So, in the physical relationship, one gradually notices, the human being becomes deficient. But I don't wish for anything that I can no longer be…
>
> The fact that I don't see you, even though I'm looking at you, I have long since accepted. It makes no sense to resist it, right. You can only accept what is, just as it is. To indulge in sorrow for even 5 minutes, that is really wasted time."

13.13 The Door Opens Inward

Yet, Count Dürckheim does not experience his life as a torture at all. He does not struggle with his situation:

> **Interview**
>
> "So for me, life becomes richer every day, because it somehow always has more backgrounds that one can perceive and discover. So I wouldn't say: I have lived enough now, I can die. I always have the feeling that something new is added. One gift simply follows the other, in what you can still experience about yourself in terms of depth dimensions: The joy of life. I like to live."

13.14 Daily Routine

That's why his daily routine looks like it did in the last 10 years before:

> **Interview**
>
> "Every day, at exactly 7 o'clock, I am in a meditation room with some people who gather there with me and sit in absolute silence from 7–8 o'clock. That's how the day starts.
>
> And then come the office hours. That means, one person after another comes to me for therapy sessions, usually 3–4 people in the morning, each about 40 minutes duration per conversation. But then there is always a time of silence. Always in the last 10 minutes, when someone comes to me, we do not speak, but we go into silence. And so every morning.
>
> The afternoon is usually the time for correspondence, the countless letters, some of which I also answer myself. Some of them are answered by my secretary independently.
>
> So the morning is the time for conversations, in the afternoon the correspondence and sometimes also another conversation."

13.15 In the Face of Death

Count Dürckheim already spoke quite openly at that time about living in the face of death and that it can reach out for him any day:

> **Interview**
>
> "I believe, the most important thing is to first accept the fact that one will die. I hope that I will be given the chance to die somewhat painlessly.
>
> Accepting death is quite natural for me. I will die one day and I wish not to have to do so in an agony of pain, so that I can consciously enter into the other life.
>
> I can never know if I won't have a heart attack tomorrow, for example. Now my heart is good in itself, and I sleep well, thank God. Perhaps because I have meditated all my life, I also have a certain stillness within me. And I often consciously enter into it. But I have no idea whether the next time I enter into the silence, I will wake up or not.
>
> But I have no fear of dying. I don't really have any special wish, only that I may be allowed to be conscious as long as possible and then to surrender myself consciously…
>
> For me, dying is the transition to another life, in which we, according to my conviction—generally I don't like to talk about what is after death, because I basically say, I can only talk about what I have experienced, and I have not yet experienced that—but in any case, for me life continues in dying—on another dimension."

Beyond right and wrong, there is a place. There we will meet. (Rumi)

13.16 Hour of Death

Karlfried Dürckheim passes away after a long period of suffering at the age of 92 on December 28, 1988, around 7 pm in Todtmoos-Rütte due to old age.

As his colleague Josef Robrecht later informed me in a phone call, Dürckheim died as he had imagined and wished: fully conscious, without pain, and almost like a gentle, accepting transition into death.

Although he could hardly see anything a few years earlier, was bedridden for half a year, probably suffered severe pain during this time and had to be cared for, he was mentally clear and prepared for his death.

Josef Robrecht, who often cared for him in his last days, reports that he frequently read texts by Meister Eckhart to him.

Dürckheim, feeling his end approaching, said goodbye to many of his colleagues—similar to C. G. Jung.

At his hour of death, his long-time companion Maria Hippius, with whom he developed initiatory therapy, was present, along with a doctor and a priest. Josef Robrecht believes that Karlfried Graf Dürckheim died as he lived, namely according to his life motto: "Become who you truly are in the depth of your being."

He is buried in the family crypt of the Dürckheim-Montmartin family in the Johanneskapelle in Steingaden.

13.17 Conclusion

Karlfried Graf Dürckheim experienced many years of wandering and transformation. Born into nobility, he survives World War I unscathed as a frontline officer. He becomes a psychology professor in Germany, engages with mysticism early on, and has enlightenment experiences ("satori"). As a Nazi diplomat, he ends up far away in Japan (perhaps because he is a "quarter Jew"), engages with Buddhism there, is interned and brought back to Germany without charge. In a small Black Forest village, he becomes a Zen master, meditation teacher, and spiritual guide. Despite (or perhaps because of) his turbulent life, he has become a very calm, meditative person who consciously, calmly, and half-blindly faces death. Not full of a thirst for adventure like C. G. Jung, but sober and enduring pain.

Further Reading

Dürckheim, Karlfried Graf: Erlebnis und Wandlung, München 1978 (O. W. Barth)
Dürckheim, Karlfried Graf: Der Ruf nach dem Meister, München 1975 (O. W. Barth)
Dürckheim, Karlfried Graf: Im Zeichen der großen Erfahrung, München 1974 (O. W. Barth)
Dürckheim, Karlfried Graf: Überweltliches Leben in der Welt, München 1972
Dürckheim, Karlfried Graf: Der Alltag als Übung: vom Weg zur Verwandlung, Bern 1983 (Huber)
Dürckheim, Karlfried Graf: Japan und die Kultur der Stille, München 1984 (Barth)
Dürckheim, Karlfried Graf: Zen und wir, München 1984 (Barth)
Dürckheim, Karlfried Graf: Wunderbare Katze und andere Zen-Texte, München 2011 (Barth)
Dürckheim, Karlfried Graf: Hara: Die energetische Mitte des Menschen, München 2012 (Barth)
Interview mit Karlfried Graf Dürckheim (1986)

14

Interlude VII: Images of Humans and Therapy Goals in Psychotherapy

Contents

Further Reading 144

> This article is about images of humanity and therapy goals. The different perspectives of various psychotherapeutic schools are compared.

Psychotherapy is still young. In its scientific form, it is only about 100 years old. There are about 600 different psychotherapy and psychotherapy-like methods: serious and less serious, elaborate and less elaborate, academically founded and offbeat. They all have founding fathers, founding mothers, founding parents. When they are elaborated, there is something like a clear philosophy, an image of humanity, a concept of disease, an inventory of methods and techniques, etc. Of course, I could only present a small selection in this book.

Nevertheless—or perhaps because of this—it is on the one hand a story of building upon each other, of integration, of merging and mutual learning from each other.

On the other hand, it is also a story of separations and demarcations, of trench warfare and mutual accusations. This is evident in various areas, e.g. in the images of humanity and therapy goals of the individual methods:

- The **psychoanalysis**—according to Sigmund Freud—has the therapy goal of making the patient capable of love and work again. Freud considers humans to be beings whose task it is to domesticate—better to cultivate—their drives: Where Id was, Ego shall be.
- Alfred Adler's **individual psychology** has set itself the goal of helping the client to take responsibility for his life, to become clear about his own life goals, to acquire the competence to achieve them, and to develop a "sense of community", i.e. the "ability to be socially connected".
- Carl Gustav Jung sees in the **analytical psychology** the task of humans to achieve "inner freedom" through "individuation". This means that in therapy one should deal with one's inadequacies ("shadow"), the opposite sex ("animus"/"anima"), and learn to allow the assimilation of the contents of the collective unconscious (archetypes).
- Wilhelm Reich sees humans primarily as biological beings. In his **orgone therapy**, he aims for the biological-energetic liberation of life energy by dissolving the muscle and character armor and restoring the full orgiastic potency ("orgasm reflex").
- Jacob L. Moreno emphasizes the social side of humans. He tries in **psychodrama** to illuminate the different aspects of a person not only theoretically but also to implement them into life and to increase his role flexibility. His credo is "Acting is more healing than talking."
- Fritz Perls aims in **Gestalt therapy** for a fulfilled, creative life in the "here and now". He is concerned with actualizing the "wisdom of the organism" and promoting personal growth in awareness.
- Karlfried Graf Dürckheim tries to give people in **initiatic therapy** assistance in dealing with the numinous, the inexplicable, the supernatural. He is concerned with mystical experience, which can give life a completely different, deeper direction: "Die before you die."

There are a multitude of ways to categorize, order, or tag the various psychotherapy methods.

The French philosopher Maryse Choisy finds an interesting image for comparing the first three major psychotherapy schools:

If someone had a car breakdown, then

- Freud would open the hood and start repairing the engine,
- Jung would run off with a canister to get gasoline, and
- Adler would bend over the map and explore the destination.

(She makes no statement about the other psychotherapy methods.)

Hilarion Petzold writes about the founders of the psychotherapy schools:

> "**Perls** often points out that **Freud** compensated for his neurosis, his phobic attitude towards direct contact, theoretically and methodically through the principle of abstinence and through analysis on the couch. Despite all exaggeration, it is made clear that great therapists have developed their method as a way of coping with personal problems, and that therapeutic methods in theory and technique are expressions of the pathological, healthy, and creative parts of their creators' personalities.
>
> **Moreno**, whose earlier expressionist poems bear megalomaniac and paranoid traits, makes himself the 'director' of the great world theater and establishes the method of psychodrama. …
>
> **Jung** integrates his fragmented, chaotic inner world and his psychosis-like episodes through his inner guru, through concepts like animus and anima, the archetypes, and techniques like active imagination.
>
> **Adler** addresses in the development of his theory his personal theme, the feeling of inferiority and the fear of the future."

Other psychotherapists make it even more headline-like. They attest:

- Sigmund Freud the will to **pleasure,**
- Alfred Adler the will to **power** and
- Victor Frankl the will to **meaning.**

Whatever the assessments of the various psychotherapy methods may look like and whatever they may say about healthy and fulfilled life and the way to die—the fundamental question is:

Is there really a connection between lifestyle and the way one dies? Or even a connection between what one achieves in life—one's "work"—and how one faces death?

There will probably be no universally valid answers to these questions and one should not expect a "art of dying" that fits all people.

At best, one will be encouraged to examine oneself and one's own lifestyle. And perhaps it is helpful to see how the great psychotherapists have dealt with it.

Further Reading

Disch, Ursula M.: Der Umgang mit dem Alter in unterschiedlichen Kulturen und Zeiten, Ingelheim 1992 (Boehringer)

Eicke, Dieter (Hrsg.): Tiefenpsychologie Bd. 1–4, Weinheim und Basel 1982 (Beltz)

Hesse, Hermann: Mit der Reife wird man jünger, Frankfurt 1990 (Insel TB)

Schreiber, Hermann: Das gute Ende, Reinbek 1996 (Rowohlt)

Zeyer, Albert: Das Geheimnis der Hundertjährigen, Zürich 1995 (Kreuz)

15

Nossrat Peseschkian (1933–2010): Death in Sleep

Contents

15.1	Origin and Extended Family	147
15.2	Kashan	147
15.3	Mother	147
15.4	Baha'i	148
15.5	School Time	149
15.6	Father	149
15.7	Music and Literature	150
15.8	Medicine	150
15.9	Wanderer between Two Worlds	151
15.10	German Language—difficult Language	151
15.11	Studies	152
15.12	Bridge Builder	152
15.13	From Body to Psyche	153
15.14	Private Practice	153
15.15	Myth Therapy and Differentiation Analysis	154
15.16	Positive Psychotherapy	154
15.17	Positum	155
15.18	Publications	156
15.19	Balance Model: Four Areas of Life	157
15.20	The Three Stages of Interaction	159
15.21	The Five-Step Treatment Strategy:	160
15.22	Use of Stories, Aphorisms, Jokes	162
15.23	The Other View of Symptoms	163
15.24	Personal Contact	164

© The Author(s), under exclusive license to Springer-Verlag GmbH, DE, part of Springer Nature 2024
W. Gross, *As One Lives, So One Dies*, https://doi.org/10.1007/978-3-662-70061-7_15

15.25	Active Until the Last Moment	165
15.26	Funeral	166
15.27	Further Development	166
15.28	Conclusion	167
Bibliography		167

> **Trailer**
>
> In this chapter, we discuss Nossrat Peseschkian, the Iranian-German founder of positive psychotherapy. He is a bridge builder not only between East and West, but also between depth psychology and behavioral therapy, and between psychiatry and psychotherapy.
>
> His method is characterized by universally understandable simplicity and humor. He died as he lived in recent years:
>
> "It is easy to take life seriously. It is difficult to take life lightly," is one of the Peseschkian phrases by which he lived. He took life lightly and simply passed away without pain in his sleep.

If you want something you've never had, you have to do something you've never done. (Nossrat Peseschkian)

> No question: Skills develop by people learning to cope with difficult—seemingly insoluble—situations. What initially seemed impossible is eventually overcome through creativity, self-discipline, and perseverance—if one does not give up. People grow from this, because there is (almost) always a solution. "Not because it is difficult do we dare not, but because we dare not, it is difficult," said the Roman philosopher Seneca over 2000 years ago.

Nossrat Peseschkian was born on June 18, 1933, in the city of Kashan, which is located in the province of Isfahan in the Iranian highlands, near the Persian salt desert.

Nossrat's childhood in old Persia (only since 1935 has it been called Iran, the "land of the Aryans", the sons of the sun) is a time of departure. Important social projects are being tackled: hospitals are being built, outpatient clinics are being established, orphanages are being set up, compulsory schooling from the age of 7 has already been introduced and the school sector is being expanded—vocational schools for technical professions and nursing are being founded, the rural population is being educated in hygiene and economic issues. In 1935, the University of Tehran was founded.

15 Nossrat Peseschkian (1933–2010): Death in Sleep

15.1 Origin and Extended Family

The extended family in which Nossrat grows up is characterized by a high degree of close, solidary group cohesion and mutual care. The family collective not only provides a certain emotional security, but on a material level it also serves as a kind of social insurance: the clan takes over guardianship in crisis situations and helps overcome financial bottlenecks. But dependence on the extended family can also quickly give rise to feelings of confinement and incapacitation.

Nossrat's father, Josef Peseschkian, was born in 1910 in Hamadan. At this time, there is famine in this area, which is why the family has to relocate to the city of Malayer—fortunately to a place where the grandfather, Soleiman, a capable businessman, had already expanded his business. Here, the grandfather also has first contacts with the Baha'i religion.

When Josef is 15 years old, his apprenticeship years begin. He gets an apprenticeship in a doctor's office and a pharmacy. He becomes a "Hakim", today he would probably be situated between pharmacist, folk doctor, healer, and naturopath. (Peseschkian translated means something like "doctor", the family name was coined by the grandfather in the 1920s, because there were no surnames in Iran until then).

In Kashan, he also meets his future wife Talat. The meeting of Nossrat's parents is recorded in the family history of the Peseschkians as a "nudge of fate": Josef actually wanted to go to Tehran, but got on the wrong bus to Kashan, where he then met his wife Talat.

Josef and Talat Peseschkian—marry in 1932 and Nossrat is born in June 1933 in Kashan.

15.2 Kashan

Kashan is famous for its "Kashan carpets" named after the city, the silk fabrics, the faience, and also for the rose water produced in the area. In a suburb of Kashan, in Fin, there is the King's Garden, where the Peseschkians often make longer trips. This King's Garden ("Baghe Shah") is a place of tolerance during Nossrat's childhood. There, Muslims, Jews, Christians, and Baha'i meet and discuss peacefully with each other.

15.3 Mother

Until the birth of his siblings, Nossrat is the undisputed prince of the Peseschkian family for the first 5 years of his life, receiving all the attention of his parents and extended family.

Nossrat's relationship with his mother Talat is described as very close and intimate. This intense mother bond was characterized more by commands than by prohibitions, in which patience, trust, and hope were central. His mother gave him sufficient freedom for autonomous development and always encouraged him to act independently and competently.

His brother Huschang is born in 1938, his sister Rezwan in 1941.

Even if one may have to relativize the idealizing oriental descriptions, Nossrat's relationship with his mother was definitely very close.

A shock for Nossrat is therefore—many years later—the sudden death of his mother on April 2, 1950, who does not survive another pregnancy. At the time of his mother's death, Nossrat has a kind of supernatural experience that almost forces him to rush home: "I felt like a knife was stabbing my heart." When he arrives, however, his mother is already dead. He later says: "One longs for a mother who died too early all one's life."

15.4 Baha'i

The Peseschkians have been Baha'i for several generations. This religion has a central significance for Nossrat, which is also reflected in his later psychotherapeutic work. The Baha'i see their faith as a "religion of unity". The twelve ethical principles of the Baha'i state:

- All of humanity should be considered as a unity.
- All people should constantly explore the truth.
- All religions have a common basis.
- Religion must be the cause of unity and harmony among people.
- Religion must be in agreement with science and reason.
- Men and women have equal rights.
- Prejudices of any kind must be discarded.
- World peace must be realized.
- Both genders should receive the best spiritual and moral education.
- Social issues must be resolved.
- A universal language and script should be introduced alongside the mother tongue.
- A world court must be established.

Baha'i are monotheists and for them, God is the highest being, creator and ruler of the entire universe. According to the Baha'i, the various religions—despite all the differences in their teachings—always proclaim only the one divine universal truth. However, all religions are dependent on the zeitgeist of their origin and the respective cultural imprint. And each divine revelation corresponds to the respective cultural and historical conditions—and not least to the intellectual and emotional comprehension of the individual generations.

The Baha'i religion emerged in the mid-19th century as an independent revelation religion from Shiite Islam. The founder Baha'u'llah (1817–1892) was persecuted and thrown into prison several times (in Baghdad, Constantinople, Akka) and exiled. At his last place of exile in Akka/Israel, the "universal house of justice" now stands and there—near Haifa—the Baha'i world community also has its central seat. Many Baha'i have lost their lives in cruel persecutions—not only in Iran.

15.5 School Time

In 1941, when Nossrat is 8 years old, the family moves to the Iranian capital, Tehran. He initially goes to a Christian missionary school there and as a Baha'i child among the many Muslim classmates, he has a hard time, as he has to endure many injustices against himself and his Baha'i friend Enayati, who is repeatedly beaten by schoolmates. Even in this difficult time, he learns to deal appropriately with conflicts and to find creative solutions. Thus, he already responds to the aggressions of his schoolmates at that time with subtly meaningful and humorous sayings.

As a 13-year-old, he attends the Khagani high school in Tehran and observes the habits and quirks of his classmates, thus conducting initial character studies and tutoring younger students.

15.6 Father

The father is described as being practically inclined on the one hand and supports his children with concrete assistance and advice. He also gives them the tools to recognize and understand natural processes and social contexts. On the other hand, he is an enthusiastic storyteller. Nossrat often raves later in life when he talks about the large family evenings of his childhood in the living room, where the father tells stories, recites poems or sometimes sings with a penetrating voice.

Nossrat adopts these characteristics to some extent and refines them in his later life.

15.7 Music and Literature

Happiness can only be held onto when it is passed on.

Nossrat is enthusiastic about music. He learns to play the violin, and singing has been part of his life since childhood, so he develops a good singing voice. Later in life, he sometimes sings the sentences while writing books or lectures before writing them down.

Above all, however, he is also fascinated by literature. He reads many of the famous Persian poets such as Saadi, Rumi, and Nizami with the same enthusiasm as the old Gathas, the holy songs of Zarathustra. He writes himself and practices in poetic competitions.

After graduating from high school, he begins a literature study in Tehran at the age of 20, in which he deals with both Persian and Western literature. The world literature he studies ranges from Goethe, Dostoevsky, Rousseau, Hemingway, Thomas Mann, Tolstoy, George Bernard Shaw to Honoré de Balzac, Oscar Wilde, and Victor Hugo. His preference for stories, which he also uses later in psychotherapy, is already evident here. Later in Germany, his enthusiasm for memorable aphorisms is deepened by the works of Wilhelm Busch, Lichtenberg, Ringelnatz, and Eugen Roth.

To balance this, he does a lot of sports already at this time, with wrestling, mountaineering, and cycling being his favorite sports.

15.8 Medicine

Besides his father, it is primarily his uncle Dr. Soleiman Berjis who introduces him to medicine. Even during his school days in Kashan, he worked in his uncle's practice, often accompanied him on house visits to patients, and even helped set up a small injection service—first in Kashan, later more professionally in Tehran. After the official recognition of his injection service, it becomes increasingly clear to Nossrat that he wants to become a doctor.

His uncle Soleiman is later, in the early 1950s, presumably (due to his Baha'i affiliation) murdered by fanatical Muslims with 81 knife stabs. An incident that even reaches the United Nations.

15.9 Wanderer between Two Worlds

In the early 1950s, there are many young Persians who go abroad to study. When Nossrat learns that studying medicine in Germany takes about 5 years—slightly shorter than in the USA and France—he immediately starts learning the German language.

Thus, Nossrat Peseschkian becomes a wanderer between two worlds. When he arrives in war-torn Freiburg in 1954 to study, he brings (at least according to the stories) a Persian carpet that initially helps him make ends meet. Later, parallel to his medical studies, he establishes an import-export company, which on the one hand imports valuable carpets to Germany and on the other hand mainly delivers medicines and medical items to Iran. Thus, in the early 1960s, even the first contact lenses from Germany are brought to Iran with his help.

Detours expand local knowledge.

15.10 German Language—difficult Language

Many anecdotes revolve around his first understanding of the German language and mentality, such as the fact that he searches in vain in the dictionary for the typical southern German filler word "gelle", which his landlady often uses. The typical Persian speech melody, the intonation, remains with him even after many years in Germany.

It also takes time to adapt to the German mentality. For example, in Persian everyday culture there is a form of politeness ("Taarof") which means that when you are offered a coffee or a piece of cake, you should first decline before accepting it.

The German mentality, on the other hand, is characterized by the fact that a rejection is taken seriously (according to the saying "who doesn't want, already has") and there is no second offer.—Thus, as an Iranian who is too polite when invited to German families, you can remain hungry.

Since he brings good social skills and abilities from Iran and quickly develops a transcultural view, such adaptation processes happen very quickly in his early days in Germany.

The world is big enough for everyone (in their own way) to be wrong.

15.11 Studies

On April 24, 1954, Peseschkian enrolls at the University of Freiburg to study human medicine. A year later, he transfers to the University of Mainz.

There in the student dormitory, he makes in-depth "transcultural experiences" with three fellow students from Spain, Africa, and Germany. His room is symbolically declared the "United Nations" room.

Own experiences are expensive, foreign experiences are valuable.

It is experiences like these that lead him to deal with the topic of cultural imprints and intercultural differences at an early stage.

A few years later, he goes to the Johann Wolfgang Goethe University in Frankfurt, where he takes his medical state examination in 1960.

After completing his medical studies, he returns to Iran in 1961 to work in a Tehran hospital. He actually wants to stay in his Iranian homeland, but there he meets Manije, a biology student, whom he marries on December 27, 1961.

The couple then goes to Germany in early 1962. Their first son Hamid is born in the same year, followed by their second son Navid in 1964.

15.12 Bridge Builder

Through his recurring travels to Iran, Peseschkian gradually becomes a bridge builder between East and West. Since he not only knows both mentalities but also lives them, he later says that he never knows exactly whether he is actually a Prussian Oriental or an Oriental Prussian.

Dr. Hamid Peseschkian, the eldest son of Nossrat and current head of the Wiesbaden Academy for Psychotherapy (WIAP), says about his father:

> **Interview**
>
> "Essentially, he was shaped by two things:
> Firstly, by this change between East and West. After all, he grew up in old Iran, still in the typical Persian culture in the 1930s and 1940s. And then in 1954, 9 years after the 2nd World War, he comes to Germany to the bombed-out Freiburg. The clash of the two cultures shaped him even then …
> Even more significant were probably his origins and his family of origin. In particular, the fact that he was a member of the Baha'i community, and these Baha'i thoughts, that man is essentially good, and this vision of the Baha'i of unity in the diversity of people, shaped him a lot. He wanted to see these cultural differences as a positive challenge."

15.13 From Body to Psyche

Nossrat initially works as a ward doctor in a facility of the state insurance institution before he deals more intensively with the subject areas of psychiatry, neurology, and psychotherapy and begins specialist training. He works at various clinics in different professional positions and receives his doctorate. In 1968 he receives his license as a specialist for nervous and mental diseases and becomes a member of the German Society for Neurology. Much later, he also becomes a specialist in psychotherapeutic medicine and for psychiatry and psychotherapy.

There are no roads, paths are created as you walk.

15.14 Private Practice

After various psychotherapeutic training and further education at home and abroad, he opens a practice with a day clinic in Wiesbaden. At the beginning, it is a completely normal medical general practice—he even initially has an X-ray machine in his practice.

But from now on, the wandering years are over, he settles down. Although he continues to travel often for lectures and seminars in the coming years, Wiesbaden is something like his "base camp" to which he always returns.

He gets to know Victor E. Frankl (logotherapy), Jacob L. Moreno (psychodrama), J. H. Schulz (autogenic training) personally and later develops close contacts with the Swiss psychiatrist Raymond Battegay and the Italian psychoanalyst Gaetano Benedetti.

Although Peseschkian understands himself and his work as depth psychology-based psychotherapy, he already has in his practice the employee Hans Deidenbach, who brings the pragmatism of behavior therapy into the psychotherapeutic work. Thus, Benedetti already stated in 1977 that "positive psychotherapy is a remarkable synthesis of psychodynamic and behavior-related elements and thus makes a significant contribution to the unified relationships within psychotherapy".

15.15 Myth Therapy and Differentiation Analysis

In addition to his practice, Peseschkian gradually begins with psychotherapeutic theory development and writes his first books in German. His son, Hamid Peseschkian, tells me in conversation:

> **Interview**
>
> "It wasn't that he wanted to strategically develop a new psychotherapy method from the start, but it more or less resulted. He does come from psychoanalysis, but in many places—e.g. with its strict abstinence requirement—it was simply too far away from everyday life. So he offered his patients the opportunity to have drinks during the sessions: a sacrilege for psychoanalysts ... Because of this and because of his origin, he was considered an exotic by some psychoanalytic colleagues. In addition, he was just as influenced by the pragmatic approach of behavior therapy as by the humanistic methods, whose image of man (that man is good at his core) had many similarities with his Baha'i view."

It is said among the Baha'is:

> *Consider man as a mine, rich in gems of inestimable value. Only education can cause it to reveal its treasures and humanity can benefit from it. (Bahá'u'lláh)*

The goal of psychotherapy is therefore to find, grind and refine the gems that are hidden in every person, so that they sparkle. Peseschkian sees this as the basis of his psychotherapeutic work. Added to this is the central factor of the transcultural perspective. Thus, a theoretical and methodological framework for his form of psychotherapy gradually matures.

Through the "myth therapy" (an idea that came to him because of his frequent use of stories in psychotherapy) and the "differentiation analysis" (from which the differentiation analytical inventory, DAI, developed), the "positive psychotherapy" developed from 1977—a term that Willi Köhler, his editor at Fischer-Verlag, found.

15.16 Positive Psychotherapy

So it can be said: The positive psychotherapy (PP) belongs to the humanistic and transcultural psychodynamic psychotherapies and also integrates systemic, psychodramatic, conversational psychotherapeutic and behavioral therapeutic elements. The basis is the positive image of humanity, which is the starting point of a resource-oriented, salutogenic and goal-oriented approach.

The goals of positive psychotherapy are the development of a positive approach in psychotherapy and the promotion of intercultural understanding. In this context, Peseschkian integrates methods and techniques from various therapy schools. In modern terms, this would be called benchmarking: adopting the best from all methods and integrating them into one's own therapy school.

From 1976 he is a lecturer at the Academy for Medical Continuing and Further Education of the Hessian Medical Association and from 1979 he also receives the authorization for further education in psychotherapy there.

Above all, however, he is also keen on scientific recognition of positive psychotherapy. In a study started in 1995 with about 300 patients, he was able to demonstrate the effectiveness of positive psychotherapy for various diseases. He also publishes (together with his colleague Hans Deidenbach) a questionnaire: "Wiesbaden Inventory for Positive Psychotherapy and Family Therapy WIPPF". An international version of the WIPPF is later developed by his colleagues and translated into several languages.

Although some psychoanalytic colleagues contemptuously call him the "storyteller", positive psychotherapy and Nossrat Peseschkian became known in the 1980s primarily through the use of stories, oriental fairy tales and wisdoms from various cultures in psychotherapy.

Sometimes his "positive psychotherapy" is also confused with Seligmann's "positive psychology" and the two gray psycho eminences engage in—albeit only at the level of correspondence—cockfights as to who has the first right to the term "positive" in connection with "psycho". (Peseschkian later sent me part of the correspondence between the two).

15.17 Positum

A central term in positive psychotherapy is the Latin term "positum". This does not mean looking at life through rose-colored glasses, but positum means seeing the "actual", the "real", the "whole"—i.e., light and shadow, the good and the problematic sides. Since traditional psychotherapy methods still focus on the problems, limitations and symptoms of patients, PP, in contrast, emphasizes the abilities and strengths of the patient.

In 1977, Peseschkian becomes president of the newly founded "German Society for Positive Psychotherapy" (DGPP) and editor of the *Journal for Positive Psychotherapy*. Since 1990, he has been working in working groups of the EAP on a European harmonization of psychotherapeutic training standards. The training in positive psychotherapy is certified by the "European Association for Psychotherapy" (EAP) as a Europe-wide psychotherapy method and as scientifically based.

> **Interview**
>
> "He was indeed a 'leader', a real figure of authority," Hamid Peseschkian tells me in an interview, "with the necessary narcissism but also the charisma. He could inspire and inspire people. He was goal-oriented, diligent and knew what he wanted. ... As a father, he was—as was customary at the time—a real head of the family, whom we naturally respected. He was not overly strict or demanding. ... I had a beautiful childhood. ... Our house was liberal and open."

And he was so open not only within the family, but also towards his patients. Hamid remembers the many late-night phone calls his father had with patients, or an incident on New Year's Eve when a patient rang the Peseschkians' doorbell because she had been thrown out of the apartment by her husband. Since she had nowhere else to go, a blanket was spread out for her in the living room, where the patient spent the night and later welcomed the New Year with the Peseschkians.

In 2000, Peseschkian founded the "Wiesbaden Academy for Psychotherapy" (WIAP) as a training center for psychological psychotherapists and KJPs. It is recognized by the state and subsequently becomes one of the leading depth psychological training and further education institutes in Germany.

15.18 Publications

It is easy to take life hard, but it is hard to take life easy.

Peseschkian travels to over 70 countries to conduct seminars, give lectures, establish institutes or give interviews. Over the years, this is supplemented by over 240 professional articles and almost 30 books, which have been translated into many languages—including textbooks (*Positive Psychotherapy, Positive Family Therapy, Psychosomatics and Positive Psychotherapy*), but also popular books in which the stories and wisdoms of life are in the foreground. The book *The Merchant and the Parrot* becomes a longseller in

Germany and is translated into more than 20 languages. In this way, he has built up a worldwide sphere of influence.

Here, Nossrat's wish to write from his youth is also fulfilled. And indeed, over the course of his life, he has developed the ability to translate the complexity of the human psyche into simple models that anyone can understand. His balance model is the most famous of these.

15.19 Balance Model: Four Areas of Life

According to the Balance Model by Peseschkian, one can say: The healthy identity of a person rests on four areas of life. These 4 life areas are usually represented in a rhombus (Fig. 15.1):

In detail, the **areas of life** mean the following:

1. **Body, Health**

This is about the relationship to one's own body. Do you use it only as a "performance machine" that has to function and nothing else? What are your own physical strengths and weaknesses? What do you do for and against your body? How does the body deal with stress? What does it signal with diseases?

How can you relax best?

The emotional world also plays a central role: Do you perceive your feelings and take them seriously? Can you still express them, or do you deny, block them in such a way that there is a risk that they will eventually thwart your plans?

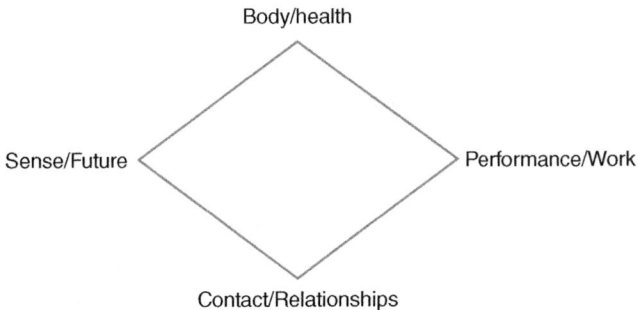

Fig. 15.1 Areas of Life

2. Work, Performance

This area is about taking a closer look at your own professional everyday life and making an actual-target analysis. What does the professional situation look like at the moment, and how would you actually like it to be? What professional goals do you have for now and the next few years? What things at the current workplace make you satisfied, and how can you get more of them? Are there perhaps structures and factors that you would like to change (and that can be changed) because you can be more satisfied and also more efficient with them? It is also about personal time structure: Isn't there more to life than increasing speed and efficiency?

3. Contact, Social Relationships

You can divide this third area again (according to the motto: Blood is thicker than water) into

a) **Partnership and Family**
These are "reprocessing plants"—but they are more than that. This pillar is about questions like: Are you satisfied with the current situation in your own relationship or do you want to change something? How much time do you spend on partnership, family? Is that enough? What about family planning? Desire for children? And what does my partner actually want? Or do you prefer to stay alone?

b) **Social Relationships, Circle of Friends, Social Commitment**
How many people do you know at all and how many of them would you call **acquaintances** and how many **friends** you can really rely on? Are there enough contacts that have nothing to do with work? What do you gain from your social relationships and what do you wish for the future? What are you socially committed to or where would you like to get involved?

4. System of Meaning (Philosophy, Religion…), Future Orientation

The last area deals with values and ideals, with what you really believe in, what is really important to you. This can be a self-made or adopted value system off the shelf, a religion, a philosophical system. If you leave the daily business outside and focus on the future: What (long-term) meaning do you see in life? Or what meaning do you give it? Where do I come from? Where am I going? What am I supposed to do here? What do I want here? Where do I want to go? What should my future look like?

Peseschkian is clear that in different phases of life, the individual areas of life are in the foreground or are subject to stress in different ways. Therefore, a precise individual analysis is necessary for each patient. While in youth, partnership, love, sexuality, and circle of friends are usually at the center of attention, in early adulthood the topic is profession and career, and afterwards perhaps starting a family, and later (or in crises) it is questions of meaning that are in the foreground.

Of course, it is good if all four areas are always stable and in balance:

This means that if you keep these four areas in mind despite your professional tension and do something to stabilize them, these are not just "psycho games", but you are doing something for your long-term development and integrating it into your own life planning. You divide your forces and develop from a short-term sprinter to a marathon runner. Because it is good to practice in the long distances and to endure both dry spells and difficult situations, which are becoming more and more frequent today.

In the end, it's about how and for what purpose I use my lifetime: How do I manage to find the right balance between external success and inner fulfillment for me?

Finally, it becomes particularly problematic when fewer than three areas have sufficient long-term stability. A healthy and satisfying life over a long period is then certainly difficult. According to Peseschkian, it is therefore important to keep life in balance, in which all four areas receive the appropriate attention and energy. That's why it's called the balance model.

15.20 The Three Stages of Interaction

Another good example of Peseschkian's ability to simplify complex issues such as communication and relationships—especially in psychotherapy—are the three stages of interaction. Because in essence, any type of (therapeutic) relationship can be divided into three phases:

- **Connection:** "Good day"

  This is about establishing a therapeutic working alliance, a sustainable emotional relationship, in which trust in the competence of the therapist is paramount. Commonalities and bonding are important—in the psychoanalytic understanding, this is the establishment of the transference and countertransference relationship.

- **Differentiation:** "How are you?"

  This is certainly the main part of the psychotherapeutic work. Here, it is less about the emotional side of the relationship, but rather about bringing the objective data to the forefront: diagnosis, anamnesis, the development of symptoms need to be perceived and differentiated. But also new (solution) strategies should develop.

- **Separation:** "Goodbye"

  The goal here is to implement the insights from psychotherapy in everyday life, to develop autonomy, to separate and also to restore the willingness for new connection.

15.21 The Five-Step Treatment Strategy:

In the psychotherapeutic process, this is concretely reflected in the 5-step approach of positive Psychotherapy:

1. **Observation/Differentiation**

    For Peseschkian, after establishing a viable therapeutic working alliance (see above), this involves the unbiased situational analysis of the patient. The patient should describe as openly as possible how he experiences his situation. The goal here for the **psychotherapist** is to achieve an unbiased perception of the patient, a kind of "beginner's mind" combined with active listening. It is about collecting information, with an appropriate proximity-distance regulation. This requires openness, awareness, sensitivity, patience, time…

    For **patients**, the central feeling is to be accepted and understood, ("being able to say everything"), the gradual development of perception and differentiation ability. His subjective views of problems and desires should be able to be expressed and first insights into their function should become understandable.

When you're up to your neck in water,
you shouldn't hang your head.

2. **Inventory**
   For the PT, this means: asking without judgment, "sorting", order, structure, function of the symptom. Tenor: Many things are difficult before they become easy.
   The psychotherapist must be aware of where he sets the focus: How deep do I go? How far do I delve (now) into the life story? What can I expect from the patient? Initial hypotheses on the origin of the problems: "cause concept", transference/countertransference.

3. **Situational Encouragement**
   While the first two stages have a more depth-psychological background, situational encouragement involves a more behavior-therapeutic-pragmatic approach.
   Self-help and resource activation of the patient (What did I do right in similar situations in the past? What worked—what didn't?), giving hope without creating illusions, and direct implementation are the goal. Ideally, the patient takes something from each session that he can directly try out and implement in everyday life.
   The patient should search for his abilities, his healthy parts, and successes in previous conflict resolutions.

   There is no elevator to happiness.
   You have to take the stairs.

4. **Verbalization**
   In this phase, the PT should provide guidance for the concretization and development of the patient's communicative abilities. It's about "clarification". The patient should perceive and express the open conflicts and problems in the four areas of life (balance model). The goal is a positive self-understanding. Motto: "The pessimist sees a problem in every opportunity, the optimist sees an opportunity in every problem."
   In this way, the patient's personal responsibility should be strengthened.

   You can't give life more days,
   but you can give the day more life.

5. **Goal Expansion**
   What else needs to be done? What's next? What can I transfer from what I've learned so far to other areas of life? Ideas…
   "And tomorrow?" "What are your goals for the next 3–5 years?" "What will you do when you no longer have complaints and problems?"

Trust: Confidence in one's own abilities and the future: Autonomy and detachment.

Don't let yourself go—go yourself.

What looks somewhat schematic here, Peseschkian has of course individualized and adapted in the concrete psychotherapeutic approach to the respective situation of the patient. Because the goal of Peseschkian and positive psychotherapy is from the beginning not the creation of dependency, but self-help and self-responsibility: You can only do it yourself—but often not alone. One of Peseschkian's favorite quotes was:

If you need a helping hand, look for it at the end of your arm.

Not only for the establishment of self-responsibility did he like to use stories, parables, proverbs, and even jokes.

15.22 Use of Stories, Aphorisms, Jokes

There is a beautiful story about why the use of stories often proves to be useful. It is called **Truth and Parable:**

> **Interview**
>
> "Once Truth and Parable met.
> While the Parable came whistling in colorful clothes, full of energy, fun and radiating joy of life, the Truth, on the other hand, trudged along grumpily, depressed, in a bad mood and serious.
> The Parable asked the Truth: 'What's wrong with you? You don't seem to be too happy—why are you living so listlessly?'
> The Truth replied: 'Nobody is interested in me and nobody wants to hear what I have to tell them—how could I have fun and feel joy of life.'
> The Parable answered: 'Oh, if that's the case: I'd be happy to give you some of my colorful clothes. Then people will be interested in you.'
> When the Truth had put on the colorful clothes of the Parable, she was welcomed by the people and received with interest."

Stories, narratives and aphorisms—as Peseschkian found out—can have many functions. The most important are:

- They facilitate a change of perspective and help to break away from old, familiar patterns of thought.
- They provoke a different viewpoint and/or a (internal) change of location.
- Sometimes they are a regression aid.
- They are diagnostic tools ("How do you understand this story?").
- They symbolize and serve as a mirror function, a model function or the function of a counter-concept for the patient.
- They are mediators between the therapist and the patient.
- They function as memory aids and have (sometimes) a depot effect.
- They encourage the use of one's own imagination.
- They help to break down prejudices and resentments.
- They contribute to a change in consciousness.

15.23 The Other View of Symptoms

Everyone is wise: one before—the other after.

The goal of using stories and life wisdom is to develop a creative imagination at the individual level and to help the patient to a different perspective on the symptoms. After all, a mental illness often goes hand in hand with a narrowed view and the opening of these blinkers is—according to Peseschkian—a first step towards change—both in terms of inner attitude and behavior.

Examples:

- **Fear:** One can see fear as the inability to face difficult situations, or as the ability to avoid threatening situations.
- **Depression** can be described as a feeling of oppression and passivity or as the ability to react with deep emotionality to conflicts.
- **Sleep disorder** can be seen as the ability to be vigilant and to get by with little sleep.
- **Frigidity** as the ability to say no through the body.
- **Anorexia** is also the ability to get by with little food.
- etc.

Of course, one must be careful that the patient does not take such an interpretation the wrong way: The feeling of not being taken seriously with his symptoms, or the interpretation of being insulted or belittled, are dangerous. But after the first "healing confusion", the penny usually drops: Because through this approach, an internal change of location often happens—both in the patient himself and often also in the environment. The patient thus experiences incidentally that his complaints are also signals to bring four areas of his life into order.

No one can be happy without his consent
(Mark Twain)

15.24 Personal Contact

When I personally met Nossrat Peseschkian in 2003 (we both gave a lecture in a Westphalian clinic), he was a man well-known in professional circles—albeit not without controversy. I had been reading his books—especially those with the oriental stories—since the mid-1980s. Even then, I was impressed by his casualness and presence. I never had the impression that he was under stress.

From 2005–2020, I conducted seminars at the Wiesbaden Academy for Psychotherapy (WIAP), which he founded and has since handed over to his son Hamid—even if he remains the "Spiritus Rector".

While Hamid takes over the institute's management from his father, the younger son Navid takes over his father's health insurance approval and practices as a specialist in child, adolescent, and adult psychiatry.

Most of the time I know him, Nossrat seems to me like someone who is full of life. He always has an appropriate quote or a casual saying on his lips. Contact with him is relaxed and open. He is generous and giving. For many of his students, he is a kind of positive father figure.

Only in recent years did I learn that he has heart problems. It is probably the first time in his life that he had to cancel a seminar in Vienna in 2001 due to a heart attack, which is said to have been very upsetting for him. He gets a stent inserted. It goes on. When he is admitted to a hospital in Stuttgart (around 2005) probably due to a minor stroke, he discharges himself ("at his own risk" as it is so nicely put) to give a lecture there. Immediately afterwards, he returns repentantly to the clinic for further treatment.

Forgetfulness is the ability to enjoy the space between memories.

The seminars he conducts also become difficult at times. "Sometimes he was hard to stop," says Hamid, his son:

Interview

"Even though he had these heart problems, he was basically relatively healthy for his age. As far as I know, he didn't take any medication. His diet was normal and since we Baha'is don't drink alcohol, his health was essentially fine. ... He did his gymnastics every day and went for walks relatively often and his enthusiasm remained until the end. He was a 'survivor' and had many more ideas and projects."

Hope is not the conviction that something will turn out well, but the certainty that something makes sense—no matter how it turns out. (Vaclav Havel)

15.25 Active Until the Last Moment

This includes that he discussed further professional projects with Birgit W. and Gunter H. at dinner until 10 pm just a few hours before his death. After a phone call with Ines S., an Austrian psychotherapist, he goes to sleep. Shortly after 1 am, his wife Manije wakes up. When she returns from the toilet, she hears that her husband is no longer breathing and notices that his body is slowly getting cold.

Nossrat Peseschkian died at the age of 78, essentially in his sleep—without noticeable cramps and pain, he was apparently able to let go easily.

It is April 27, 2010, around 2 am, when Manije calls her two sons. They are with her shortly afterwards and all the necessary steps are initiated.

The next morning, the closest relatives are called first, and then all those from the family and circle of friends who should know first that he has died before the general public finds out.

Then come the funeral formalities that need to be prepared, and later the official announcements for the students of positive psychotherapy.

Not least because the relatives come from very far away (partly from New Zealand or Los Angeles), the funeral takes place a few days later. More than 500 people attend the funeral.

> **Interview**
>
> "His sudden death—frankly—did not completely surprise me, as he had been having heart problems for several months," Hamid Peseschkian tells me in an interview. "I believe he died as a content man—even though he still had a lot planned."

In his book article "Everyone Wants to Go to Heaven, But No One Wants to Die" (Burbach/Heckmann, p. 219), Nossrat Peseschkian quoted Baha'u'llah shortly before his death:

"Examine yourself every day before you are held accountable. For death comes unexpectedly."

15.26 Funeral

Since for the Baha'is, dying is a transition to another state of being, death is not only full of grief, sorrow, and pain. So one can say, Nossrat Peseschkian left as he lived the last years—simple and light. "Don't be sad that it's over," he sometimes said, "be glad that it happened".

And this also fit: According to the Baha'is, the dead should not be driven hundreds of kilometers around, but should be buried near the place of death. The Peseschkian family home is just 500 m from the cemetery where Nossrat is buried in an earth grave.

15.27 Further Development

Even after his death, the development of positive psychotherapy continues. His wife Manije (who dies only 10 years later) and his sons Hamid and Navid take over the further development and professionalization of positive psychotherapy. The fact that their children are also in training to become doctors and psychologists, Nossrat has probably laid the foundation for a dynasty of doctors/psychotherapists.

The "International Academy of Positive and Transcultural Psychotherapy" (IAPP), founded in 2005, which supports publications and non-profit and scientific projects, and the "World Association for Positive Psychotherapy" (WAPP), which has existed since 1994, guide the international activities. To this day, seminars, further education and lectures on positive psychotherapy are held in over 80 countries with more than 100,000 participants. The WAPP's curricula for the basic and master's degree programs in PP have been increasingly professionalized and standardized worldwide in recent years.

In 2021, the "World Association of Positive and Transcultural Psychotherapy (WAPP)" has over 2000 members. So far, the WAPP has held six world congresses of positive psychotherapy. In over 20 countries with 40 centers and institutes, almost 150 trainers teach and practice positive psychotherapy—and there are now several national PP associations (Germany, Ukraine, Bulgaria, Turkey, Romania, Kosovo, Ethiopia etc.). In some cases, PP further education can also be found in university curricula (e.g. in Russia, Turkey, Bulgaria, Bolivia).

If Nossrat Peseschkian could see what his project of positive psychotherapy has become, he would probably be proud of it today.

15.28 Conclusion

Nossrat Peseschkian, the transcultural bridge builder between East and West, between depth psychology therapy and behavior therapy, died as he lived in his last years. "It is easy to take life hard. It is hard to take life easy," is also one of the Peseschkian phrases he lived by. He took life easy and simply left without pain.

Bibliography

Burbach, Christiane, Heckmann, Friedrich: Übergänge - Annäherung an das eigene Sterben, Göttingen 2010 (Vandenhoeck + Ruprecht)

Peseschkian, Hamid, Remers, Arno: Positive Psychotherapie, München 2013 (Reinhardt)

Peseschkian, Nossrat: Psychotherapie des Alltagslebens, Frankfurt am Main 1974 (S. Fischer)

Peseschkian, Nossrat: Positive Psychotherapie. Frankfurt am Main 1977 (S. Fischer)

Peseschkian, Nossrat: Positive Familientherapie, Frankfurt am Main 1980 (S. Fischer)

Peseschkian, Nossrat: Der Kaufmann und der Papagei. Orientalische Geschichten als Medien in der Psychotherapie. Mit Fallbeispielen zur Erziehung und Selbsthilfe. Frankfurt am Main; 30. Auflage (S. Fischer)

Peseschkian, Nossrat: Psychosomatik und Positive Psychotherapie. 8. Auflage, Frankfurt am Main 2005 (S. Fischer)

Peseschkian, Nossrat: Der nackte Kaiser oder: Wie man die Seele der Kinder und Jugendlichen versteht und heilt. 2. Auflage, Frankfurt am Main 2005 (S. Fischer)

Peseschkian, Nossrat: Wenn du willst, was du noch nie gehabt hast, dann tu, was du noch nie getan hast. 14. Auflage. Freiburg 2005 (Herder)

Peseschkian, Nossrat: Glaube an Gott und binde dein Kamel fest. Warum Religion unserer Seele gut tut. Stuttgart 2008 (Kreuz)

16

Epilogue: Live Your Dying

Contents

Further Reading 173

> **Trailer**
> This Chapter is something like the conclusion, the inference, of the entire book. It is about comparing the lifestyles and styles of dying of the eight great psychotherapists presented in this book—and what this has to do with the psychotherapy method they developed.
> This contribution also deals with how we evade with our finiteness and the (more or less hidden) horror of death.

In the end, everything will be fine. If it's not fine, it's not the end yet. (Oscar Wilde)

How one has lived, so one dies—is that really so?

Does the way one has lived, what one has felt and thought, unfold and realize itself in dying? Or is it perhaps the other way around: Is the course of life unconsciously oriented towards dying? Does it have a (more or less conscious) goal? Is there such a thing as a "drive destiny"? Is perhaps everything predestined—and we can't influence it or only within very narrow limits?

But—don't all theories and concepts melt away in the face of the death of a (beloved) person and become a farce?

When comparing the different ways in which the great psychotherapists have died, it is noticeable that their dying is a continuation of their life lived up to that point. The dying fits the respective person and also the psychotherapeutic method that the person in question has developed. Thus, it is also an implementation of their image of man, their theory of man.

Can we learn a lesson from the death of the great psychotherapists—and what could it be? Let's think back:

- **Freud**, the strict, serious and composed father of psychoanalysis and his long, sorrowful and morphine-sedated path into death.
- **Adler**, the life-loving, almost hectically traveling founder of individual psychology, who unexpectedly succumbs to a heart attack without a long struggle with death.
- **Reich**, who—whether gone mad or not—has to watch in prison as his entire life's work is destroyed, and who eventually just gives up.
- **Moreno**, who sees his time as expired, lies down in bed, lets his students parade by one more time and simply stops eating in a death fast, so as not to oppose death.
- **Perls**, who his whole life emphasized the "here and now" and his individual freedom almost defiantly, dies quasi out of resistance against the sensible orders of the nurse.
- **Jung**, who in essence prepared for his death for 17 years of his life—since his accident and his near-death experiences—and who bids farewell to this world with hope for an interesting adventure.
- **Count Dürckheim**, who wanted to accept his death at any time long before, dies as he imagined: Fully conscious and sober, he accepts death.
- **Peseschkian,** the transcultural bridge builder between East and West, between depth psychology therapy and behavior therapy, died as he had lived in recent years: He took life lightly and probably fell asleep into death without pain.

In the end, there are more questions than answers. Because a final certainty about what happens when we die and what happens after death, we as living beings will not get. All information in this regard is without guarantee. All we have left is faith, hope—we will not know. We can wish for a certain death, we can expect something to happen—but at least at this point the power of our conscious will ends.

Mindful of the fact that we will all—each for himself—die: How do I actually wish to die?

- Quickly, suddenly and unexpectedly, like Alfred Adler?
- Gently sliding over in sleep, more or less, like Nossrat Peseschkian?
- Full of curiosity about the future adventure ("how wonderful"), like Carl Gustav Jung?
- Enduring the pain with morphine, like Sigmund Freud?
- Staged as a psychodrama, like Jacob L. Moreno?
- Conscious and sober like Count Dürckheim?
- In protest against the limiting reality of cancer, like Fritz Perls?
- Hardly anyone will probably wish for death in prison, as suffered by Wilhelm Reich, who ultimately died for his ideas—but who knows …

As a biological fact, death is something trivial. In death—medically "exitus"—laws are confirmed to which the entire nature is subject:

Becoming and passing away, emerging, growing, reaching the peak and then—the gradual—more or less rapid—descent, the decay, up to that qualitative leap.

The small truth has many words. The great truth has only silence. (Zen)

But there is also another side to death: The incomprehensible, the more or less hidden horror. "If we are already born—why do we have to die?", one could ask. And it is precisely this side that makes us repress death.

It is precisely the denial of death in our society that—at least in part—is responsible for many people leading an empty, meaningless life because they are not aware of their finiteness and live as if it would go on forever.

Death is not the meaningless end of human life. It is the final stage of maturity—if we understand how to see it that way. It can even become the source of meaning for our existence if we hear the radical question about the meaning of life in it and really ask ourselves this question.

"To consider that we must die makes us wise," it says in a psalm.

To consider how we will die makes us fearful. And psychotherapists—especially those who have founded their own school—are not supposed to be afraid, according to many people's opinion.

Psychotherapists and psychotherapy methods are also children of their time—even if they claim eternal values. Because it is true—no one escapes the follies of his era: What is valid today may be deceitful tomorrow and forgotten the day after. And this of course also applies to psychotherapy methods.

In the quicksand of history, one or the other psychotherapy method once praised as "new", "unique and revolutionary" may sink. But there is also the consolation of a Hungarian proverb: "The truth sometimes goes under—but it does not die."

By denying our finiteness, we also lose death as an advisor: "memento mori", remember death, is therefore the greeting formula of the members of the Christian Carthusian Order when they meet: "Remember your mortality". But in all serious spiritual and philosophical directions, the advice is similar.

"Vanitas", the vanity and transience of all earthly things, shows that man does not really have power over his life. Even for materialists who do not want or cannot adopt a religious belief system off the shelf, the question of meaning remains: Perhaps for them life has no (predetermined) meaning. But it is then also certain that one can give life a meaning (and perhaps must). And whether one takes this as a conscious task and realizes it in one's life is highly individual and varies greatly from person to person.

Since the human species has developed consciousness (whatever that exactly is), death has an unimaginable horror in it. The Danish philosopher Kierkegaard called this horror and fear the "dizziness of freedom". Probably the way people deal with the mystery of death has always been fraught with fear.—Ignoring, repressing, forgetting, veiling were and are our coping strategies. But never before have greater efforts been made to prolong life, to avoid dying, to push it back into eternity, so to speak. And it is precisely the psychotherapists, those strange magicians, who are often unconsciously blamed for having—if not immortal—at least a very special death. What is forgotten is that even great psychotherapists are not the monuments that one has of them in one's head, but people of flesh and blood. They too have a right to weaknesses—especially when it comes to dying. Because it is precisely here that it becomes apparent that these famous role models at the end of their path did not simply face death more consciously, but, like many others, had to struggle with their own inadequacies, weaknesses and doubts.

Death is inherent in life. It is not a breakdown, not a disaster.

And our life is finite. And how one deals with one's own, personal finiteness is not only a question of psychotherapy—at least if one understands it only as treatment of the sick, i.e. as healing of disease: Unless one considers death, which we all face, as a disease.

A palliative care doctor once told me: "Since death exists, it is important to cultivate dealing with it. One should not believe that life could eliminate death." As George Bernard Shaw wrote: "Do not try to live forever, you will not succeed."

And perhaps the lesson from this can be that death is always and everywhere the great equalizer—whether poor or rich, stupid or clever, whether reflective or dull, whether blonde northerner or dark-skinned African—it will hit us all and we will all experience it. What happens afterwards, we will—each for ourselves—see and experience.

More important than the question "is there life after death?" is in the end rather the question "is there life before death?"

"Carpe diem"—seize the day.

Further Reading

Eicke, Dieter (Hrsg.): Tiefenpsychologie Bd. 1–4, Weinheim und Basel 1982 (Beltz)

Keleman, Stanley: Lebe dein Sterben, Hamburg 1977 (Isko-Press)

Korp, Harald-Alexander: Am Ende ist nicht Schluss mit lustig, Gütersloh 2014 (Gütersloher Verlagshaus)

Mulford, Prentice: Unfug des Lebens und des Sterbens, Frankfurt 1977 (Fischer TB)

Schultz, Hans Jürgen (Hrsg.): Letzte Tage, Stuttgart 1983 (Kreuz)

Spiegel-Rössing, Ina, Petzold, Hilarion: Die Begleitung Sterbender – Theorie und Praxis der Thanatotherapie, Paderborn 1984 (Junfermann)

Watts, Alan: Tod, Basel 1977 (Sphinx)

Yalom, Irvin D. + Marilyn: Unzertrennlich – Über den Tod und das Leben, München 2021 (BTB)

Printed by Printforce, the Netherlands